Mometrix
TEST PREPARATION

Gastroenterology Board Exam Secrets Study Guide

DEAR FUTURE EXAM SUCCESS STORY

First of all, **THANK YOU** for purchasing Mometrix study materials!

Second, congratulations! You are one of the few determined test-takers who are committed to doing whatever it takes to excel on your exam. **You have come to the right place.** We developed these study materials with one goal in mind: to deliver you the information you need in a format that's concise and easy to use.

In addition to optimizing your guide for the content of the test, we've outlined our recommended steps for breaking down the preparation process into small, attainable goals so you can make sure you stay on track.

We've also analyzed the entire test-taking process, identifying the most common pitfalls and showing how you can overcome them and be ready for any curveball the test throws you.

Standardized testing is one of the biggest obstacles on your road to success, which only increases the importance of doing well in the high-pressure, high-stakes environment of test day. Your results on this test could have a significant impact on your future, and this guide provides the information and practical advice to help you achieve your full potential on test day.

Your success is our success

We would love to hear from you! If you would like to share the story of your exam success or if you have any questions or comments in regard to our products, please contact us at **800-673-8175** or **support@mometrix.com**.

Thanks again for your business and we wish you continued success!

Sincerely,
The Mometrix Test Preparation Team

Need more help? Check out our flashcards at:
http://MometrixFlashcards.com/Gastroenterology

Written and edited by the Mometrix Exam Secrets Test Prep Team
Printed in the United States of America

TABLE OF CONTENTS

INTRODUCTION ____ 1
SECRET KEY #1 – PLAN BIG, STUDY SMALL ____ 2
SECRET KEY #2 – MAKE YOUR STUDYING COUNT ____ 3
SECRET KEY #3 – PRACTICE THE RIGHT WAY ____ 4
SECRET KEY #4 – PACE YOURSELF ____ 6
SECRET KEY #5 – HAVE A PLAN FOR GUESSING ____ 7
TEST-TAKING STRATEGIES ____ 10
ESOPHAGUS ____ 15
STOMACH/DUODENUM ____ 22
SMALL INTESTINE ____ 35
COLON ____ 49
LIVER ____ 66
PANCREAS ____ 87
BILIARY TRACT ____ 90
HOW TO OVERCOME TEST ANXIETY ____ 92
ONLINE RESOURCES ____ 98

Introduction

Thank you for purchasing this resource! You have made the choice to prepare yourself for a test that could have a huge impact on your future, and this guide is designed to help you be fully ready for test day. Obviously, it's important to have a solid understanding of the test material, but you also need to be prepared for the unique environment and stressors of the test, so that you can perform to the best of your abilities.

For this purpose, the first section that appears in this guide is the **Secret Keys**. We've devoted countless hours to meticulously researching what works and what doesn't, and we've boiled down our findings to the five most impactful steps you can take to improve your performance on the test. We start at the beginning with study planning and move through the preparation process, all the way to the testing strategies that will help you get the most out of what you know when you're finally sitting in front of the test.

We recommend that you start preparing for your test as far in advance as possible. However, if you've bought this guide as a last-minute study resource and only have a few days before your test, we recommend that you skip over the first two Secret Keys since they address a long-term study plan.

If you struggle with **test anxiety**, we strongly encourage you to check out our recommendations for how you can overcome it. Test anxiety is a formidable foe, but it can be beaten, and we want to make sure you have the tools you need to defeat it.

Secret Key #1 – Plan Big, Study Small

There's a lot riding on your performance. If you want to ace this test, you're going to need to keep your skills sharp and the material fresh in your mind. You need a plan that lets you review everything you need to know while still fitting in your schedule. We'll break this strategy down into three categories.

Information Organization

Start with the information you already have: the official test outline. From this, you can make a complete list of all the concepts you need to cover before the test. Organize these concepts into groups that can be studied together, and create a list of any related vocabulary you need to learn so you can brush up on any difficult terms. You'll want to keep this vocabulary list handy once you actually start studying since you may need to add to it along the way.

Time Management

Once you have your set of study concepts, decide how to spread them out over the time you have left before the test. Break your study plan into small, clear goals so you have a manageable task for each day and know exactly what you're doing. Then just focus on one small step at a time. When you manage your time this way, you don't need to spend hours at a time studying. Studying a small block of content for a short period each day helps you retain information better and avoid stressing over how much you have left to do. You can relax knowing that you have a plan to cover everything in time. In order for this strategy to be effective though, you have to start studying early and stick to your schedule. Avoid the exhaustion and futility that comes from last-minute cramming!

Study Environment

The environment you study in has a big impact on your learning. Studying in a coffee shop, while probably more enjoyable, is not likely to be as fruitful as studying in a quiet room. It's important to keep distractions to a minimum. You're only planning to study for a short block of time, so make the most of it. Don't pause to check your phone or get up to find a snack. It's also important to **avoid multitasking**. Research has consistently shown that multitasking will make your studying dramatically less effective. Your study area should also be comfortable and well-lit so you don't have the distraction of straining your eyes or sitting on an uncomfortable chair.

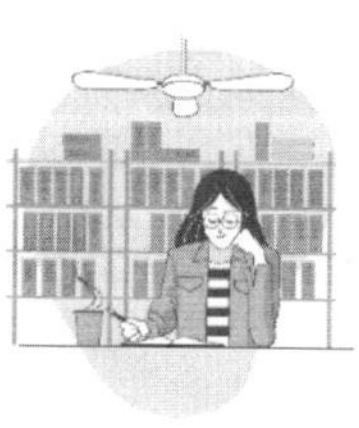

The time of day you study is also important. You want to be rested and alert. Don't wait until just before bedtime. Study when you'll be most likely to comprehend and remember. Even better, if you know what time of day your test will be, set that time aside for study. That way your brain will be used to working on that subject at that specific time and you'll have a better chance of recalling information.

Finally, it can be helpful to team up with others who are studying for the same test. Your actual studying should be done in as isolated an environment as possible, but the work of organizing the information and setting up the study plan can be divided up. In between study sessions, you can discuss with your teammates the concepts that you're all studying and quiz each other on the details. Just be sure that your teammates are as serious about the test as you are. If you find that your study time is being replaced with social time, you might need to find a new team.

Secret Key #2 – Make Your Studying Count

You're devoting a lot of time and effort to preparing for this test, so you want to be absolutely certain it will pay off. This means doing more than just reading the content and hoping you can remember it on test day. It's important to make every minute of study count. There are two main areas you can focus on to make your studying count.

Retention

It doesn't matter how much time you study if you can't remember the material. You need to make sure you are retaining the concepts. To check your retention of the information you're learning, try recalling it at later times with minimal prompting. Try carrying around flashcards and glance at one or two from time to time or ask a friend who's also studying for the test to quiz you.

To enhance your retention, look for ways to put the information into practice so that you can apply it rather than simply recalling it. If you're using the information in practical ways, it will be much easier to remember. Similarly, it helps to solidify a concept in your mind if you're not only reading it to yourself but also explaining it to someone else. Ask a friend to let you teach them about a concept you're a little shaky on (or speak aloud to an imaginary audience if necessary). As you try to summarize, define, give examples, and answer your friend's questions, you'll understand the concepts better and they will stay with you longer. Finally, step back for a big picture view and ask yourself how each piece of information fits with the whole subject. When you link the different concepts together and see them working together as a whole, it's easier to remember the individual components.

Finally, practice showing your work on any multi-step problems, even if you're just studying. Writing out each step you take to solve a problem will help solidify the process in your mind, and you'll be more likely to remember it during the test.

Modality

Modality simply refers to the means or method by which you study. Choosing a study modality that fits your own individual learning style is crucial. No two people learn best in exactly the same way, so it's important to know your strengths and use them to your advantage.

For example, if you learn best by visualization, focus on visualizing a concept in your mind and draw an image or a diagram. Try color-coding your notes, illustrating them, or creating symbols that will trigger your mind to recall a learned concept. If you learn best by hearing or discussing information, find a study partner who learns the same way or read aloud to yourself. Think about how to put the information in your own words. Imagine that you are giving a lecture on the topic and record yourself so you can listen to it later.

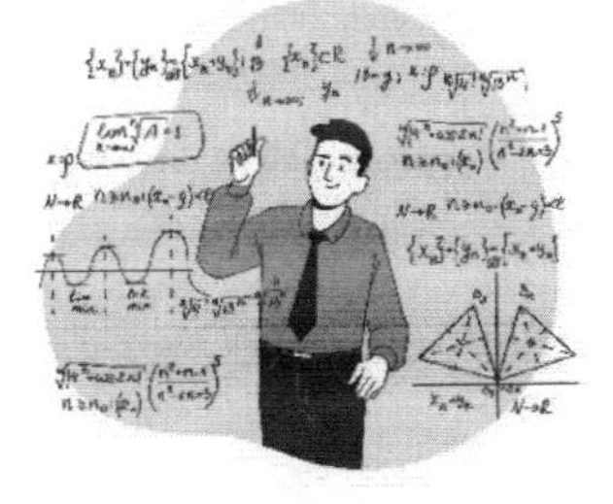

For any learning style, flashcards can be helpful. Organize the information so you can take advantage of spare moments to review. Underline key words or phrases. Use different colors for different categories. Mnemonic devices (such as creating a short list in which every item starts with the same letter) can also help with retention. Find what works best for you and use it to store the information in your mind most effectively and easily.

Secret Key #3 – Practice the Right Way

Your success on test day depends not only on how many hours you put into preparing, but also on whether you prepared the right way. It's good to check along the way to see if your studying is paying off. One of the most effective ways to do this is by taking practice tests to evaluate your progress. Practice tests are useful because they show exactly where you need to improve. Every time you take a practice test, pay special attention to these three groups of questions:

- The questions you got wrong
- The questions you had to guess on, even if you guessed right
- The questions you found difficult or slow to work through

This will show you exactly what your weak areas are, and where you need to devote more study time. Ask yourself why each of these questions gave you trouble. Was it because you didn't understand the material? Was it because you didn't remember the vocabulary? Do you need more repetitions on this type of question to build speed and confidence? Dig into those questions and figure out how you can strengthen your weak areas as you go back to review the material.

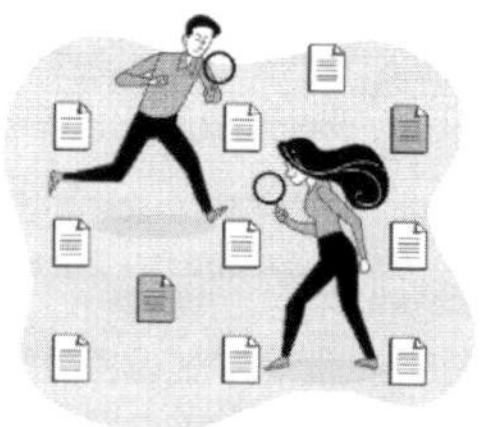

Additionally, many practice tests have a section explaining the answer choices. It can be tempting to read the explanation and think that you now have a good understanding of the concept. However, an explanation likely only covers part of the question's broader context. Even if the explanation makes perfect sense, **go back and investigate** every concept related to the question until you're positive you have a thorough understanding.

As you go along, keep in mind that the practice test is just that: practice. Memorizing these questions and answers will not be very helpful on the actual test because it is unlikely to have any of the same exact questions. If you only know the right answers to the sample questions, you won't be prepared for the real thing. **Study the concepts** until you understand them fully, and then you'll be able to answer any question that shows up on the test.

It's important to wait on the practice tests until you're ready. If you take a test on your first day of study, you may be overwhelmed by the amount of material covered and how much you need to learn. Work up to it gradually.

On test day, you'll need to be prepared for answering questions, managing your time, and using the test-taking strategies you've learned. It's a lot to balance, like a mental marathon that will have a big impact on your future. Like training for a marathon, you'll need to start slowly and work your way up. When test day arrives, you'll be ready.

Start with the strategies you've read in the first two Secret Keys—plan your course and study in the way that works best for you. If you have time, consider using multiple study resources to get different approaches to the same concepts. It can be helpful to see difficult concepts from more than one angle. Then find a good source for practice tests. Many times, the test website will suggest potential study resources or provide sample tests.

Practice Test Strategy

If you're able to find at least three practice tests, we recommend this strategy:

Untimed and Open-Book Practice

Take the first test with no time constraints and with your notes and study guide handy. Take your time and focus on applying the strategies you've learned.

Timed and Open-Book Practice

Take the second practice test open-book as well, but set a timer and practice pacing yourself to finish in time.

Timed and Closed-Book Practice

Take any other practice tests as if it were test day. Set a timer and put away your study materials. Sit at a table or desk in a quiet room, imagine yourself at the testing center, and answer questions as quickly and accurately as possible.

Keep repeating timed and closed-book tests on a regular basis until you run out of practice tests or it's time for the actual test. Your mind will be ready for the schedule and stress of test day, and you'll be able to focus on recalling the material you've learned.

Secret Key #4 – Pace Yourself

Once you're fully prepared for the material on the test, your biggest challenge on test day will be managing your time. Just knowing that the clock is ticking can make you panic even if you have plenty of time left. Work on pacing yourself so you can build confidence against the time constraints of the exam. Pacing is a difficult skill to master, especially in a high-pressure environment, so **practice is vital**.

Set time expectations for your pace based on how much time is available. For example, if a section has 60 questions and the time limit is 30 minutes, you know you have to average 30 seconds or less per question in order to answer them all. Although 30 seconds is the hard limit, set 25 seconds per question as your goal, so you reserve extra time to spend on harder questions. When you budget extra time for the harder questions, you no longer have any reason to stress when those questions take longer to answer.

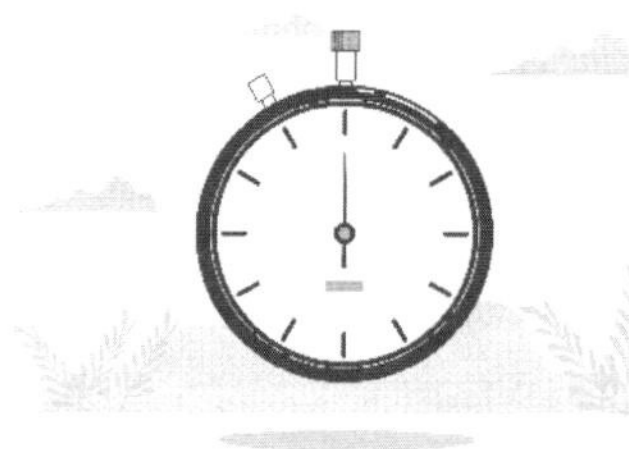

Don't let this time expectation distract you from working through the test at a calm, steady pace, but keep it in mind so you don't spend too much time on any one question. Recognize that taking extra time on one question you don't understand may keep you from answering two that you do understand later in the test. If your time limit for a question is up and you're still not sure of the answer, mark it and move on, and come back to it later if the time and the test format allow. If the testing format doesn't allow you to return to earlier questions, just make an educated guess; then put it out of your mind and move on.

On the easier questions, be careful not to rush. It may seem wise to hurry through them so you have more time for the challenging ones, but it's not worth missing one if you know the concept and just didn't take the time to read the question fully. Work efficiently but make sure you understand the question and have looked at all of the answer choices, since more than one may seem right at first.

Even if you're paying attention to the time, you may find yourself a little behind at some point. You should speed up to get back on track, but do so wisely. Don't panic; just take a few seconds less on each question until you're caught up. Don't guess without thinking, but do look through the answer choices and eliminate any you know are wrong. If you can get down to two choices, it is often worthwhile to guess from those. Once you've chosen an answer, move on and don't dwell on any that you skipped or had to hurry through. If a question was taking too long, chances are it was one of the harder ones, so you weren't as likely to get it right anyway.

On the other hand, if you find yourself getting ahead of schedule, it may be beneficial to slow down a little. The more quickly you work, the more likely you are to make a careless mistake that will affect your score. You've budgeted time for each question, so don't be afraid to spend that time. Practice an efficient but careful pace to get the most out of the time you have.

Secret Key #5 – Have a Plan for Guessing

When you're taking the test, you may find yourself stuck on a question. Some of the answer choices seem better than others, but you don't see the one answer choice that is obviously correct. What do you do?

The scenario described above is very common, yet most test takers have not effectively prepared for it. Developing and practicing a plan for guessing may be one of the single most effective uses of your time as you get ready for the exam.

In developing your plan for guessing, there are three questions to address:

- When should you start the guessing process?
- How should you narrow down the choices?
- Which answer should you choose?

When to Start the Guessing Process

Unless your plan for guessing is to select C every time (which, despite its merits, is not what we recommend), you need to leave yourself enough time to apply your answer elimination strategies. Since you have a limited amount of time for each question, that means that if you're going to give yourself the best shot at guessing correctly, you have to decide quickly whether or not you will guess.

Of course, the best-case scenario is that you don't have to guess at all, so first, see if you can answer the question based on your knowledge of the subject and basic reasoning skills. Focus on the key words in the question and try to jog your memory of related topics. Give yourself a chance to bring the knowledge to mind, but once you realize that you don't have (or you can't access) the knowledge you need to answer the question, it's time to start the guessing process.

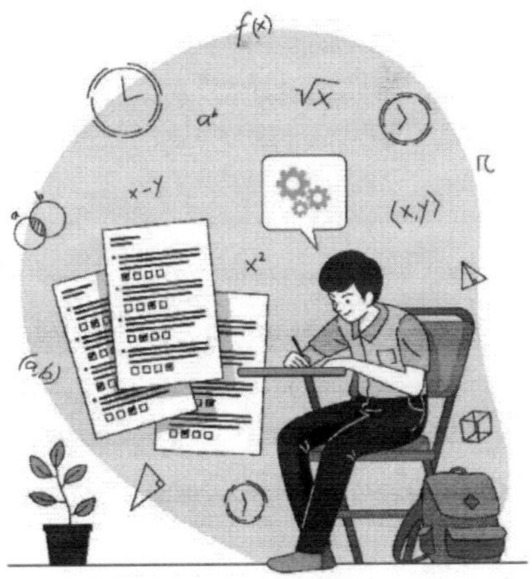

It's almost always better to start the guessing process too early than too late. It only takes a few seconds to remember something and answer the question from knowledge. Carefully eliminating wrong answer choices takes longer. Plus, going through the process of eliminating answer choices can actually help jog your memory.

Summary: Start the guessing process as soon as you decide that you can't answer the question based on your knowledge.

How to Narrow Down the Choices

The next chapter in this book (**Test-Taking Strategies**) includes a wide range of strategies for how to approach questions and how to look for answer choices to eliminate. You will definitely want to read those carefully, practice them, and figure out which ones work best for you. Here though, we're going to address a mindset rather than a particular strategy.

Your odds of guessing an answer correctly depend on how many options you are choosing from.

Number of options left	5	4	3	2	1
Odds of guessing correctly	20%	25%	33%	50%	100%

You can see from this chart just how valuable it is to be able to eliminate incorrect answers and make an educated guess, but there are two things that many test takers do that cause them to miss out on the benefits of guessing:

- Accidentally eliminating the correct answer
- Selecting an answer based on an impression

We'll look at the first one here, and the second one in the next section.

To avoid accidentally eliminating the correct answer, we recommend a thought exercise called **the $5 challenge**. In this challenge, you only eliminate an answer choice from contention if you are willing to bet $5 on it being wrong. Why $5? Five dollars is a small but not insignificant amount of money. It's an amount you could afford to lose but wouldn't want to throw away. And while losing $5 once might not hurt too much, doing it twenty times will set you back $100. In the same way, each small decision you make—eliminating a choice here, guessing on a question there—won't by itself impact your score very much, but when you put them all together, they can make a big difference. By holding each answer choice elimination decision to a higher standard, you can reduce the risk of accidentally eliminating the correct answer.

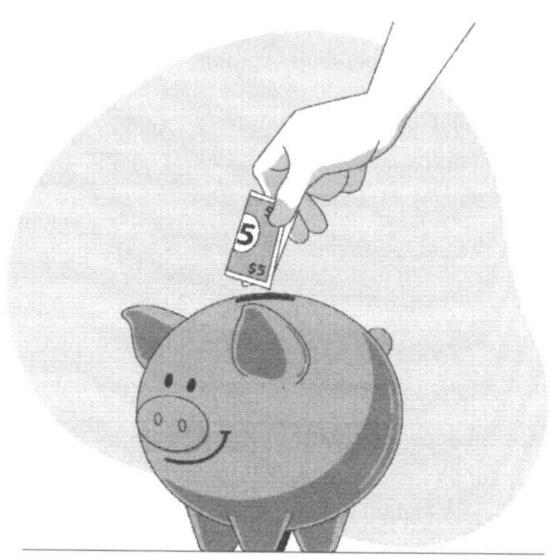

The $5 challenge can also be applied in a positive sense: If you are willing to bet $5 that an answer choice *is* correct, go ahead and mark it as correct.

Summary: Only eliminate an answer choice if you are willing to bet $5 that it is wrong.

Which Answer to Choose

You're taking the test. You've run into a hard question and decided you'll have to guess. You've eliminated all the answer choices you're willing to bet $5 on. Now you have to pick an answer. Why do we even need to talk about this? Why can't you just pick whichever one you feel like when the time comes?

The answer to these questions is that if you don't come into the test with a plan, you'll rely on your impression to select an answer choice, and if you do that, you risk falling into a trap. The test writers know that everyone who takes their test will be guessing on some of the questions, so they intentionally write wrong answer choices to seem plausible. You still have to pick an answer though, and if the wrong answer choices are designed to look right, how can you ever be sure that you're not falling for their trap? The best solution we've found to this dilemma is to take the decision out of your hands entirely. Here is the process we recommend:

Once you've eliminated any choices that you are confident (willing to bet $5) are wrong, select the first remaining choice as your answer.

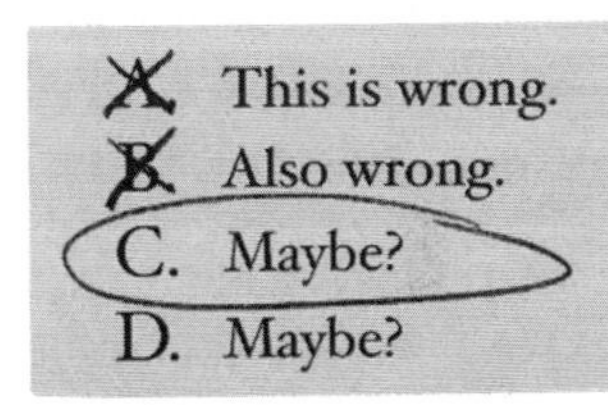

Whether you choose to select the first remaining choice, the second, or the last, the important thing is that you use some preselected standard. Using this approach guarantees that you will not be enticed into selecting an answer choice that looks right, because you are not basing your decision on how the answer choices look.

This is not meant to make you question your knowledge. Instead, it is to help you recognize the difference between your knowledge and your impressions. There's a huge difference between thinking an answer is right because of what you know, and thinking an answer is right because it looks or sounds like it should be right.

Summary: To ensure that your selection is appropriately random, make a predetermined selection from among all answer choices you have not eliminated.

Test-Taking Strategies

This section contains a list of test-taking strategies that you may find helpful as you work through the test. By taking what you know and applying logical thought, you can maximize your chances of answering any question correctly!

It is very important to realize that every question is different and every person is different: no single strategy will work on every question, and no single strategy will work for every person. That's why we've included all of them here, so you can try them out and determine which ones work best for different types of questions and which ones work best for you.

Question Strategies

⊘ Read Carefully

Read the question and the answer choices carefully. Don't miss the question because you misread the terms. You have plenty of time to read each question thoroughly and make sure you understand what is being asked. Yet a happy medium must be attained, so don't waste too much time. You must read carefully and efficiently.

⊘ Contextual Clues

Look for contextual clues. If the question includes a word you are not familiar with, look at the immediate context for some indication of what the word might mean. Contextual clues can often give you all the information you need to decipher the meaning of an unfamiliar word. Even if you can't determine the meaning, you may be able to narrow down the possibilities enough to make a solid guess at the answer to the question.

⊘ Prefixes

If you're having trouble with a word in the question or answer choices, try dissecting it. Take advantage of every clue that the word might include. Prefixes can be a huge help. Usually, they allow you to determine a basic meaning. *Pre-* means before, *post-* means after, *pro-* is positive, *de-* is negative. From prefixes, you can get an idea of the general meaning of the word and try to put it into context.

⊘ Hedge Words

Watch out for critical hedge words, such as *likely, may, can, often, almost, mostly, usually, generally, rarely,* and *sometimes.* Question writers insert these hedge phrases to cover every possibility. Often an answer choice will be wrong simply because it leaves no room for exception. Be on guard for answer choices that have definitive words such as *exactly* and *always.*

⊘ Switchback Words

Stay alert for *switchbacks.* These are the words and phrases frequently used to alert you to shifts in thought. The most common switchback words are *but, although,* and *however.* Others include *nevertheless, on the other hand, even though, while, in spite of, despite,* and *regardless of.* Switchback words are important to catch because they can change the direction of the question or an answer choice.

☑ Face Value

When in doubt, use common sense. Accept the situation in the problem at face value. Don't read too much into it. These problems will not require you to make wild assumptions. If you have to go beyond creativity and warp time or space in order to have an answer choice fit the question, then you should move on and consider the other answer choices. These are normal problems rooted in reality. The applicable relationship or explanation may not be readily apparent, but it is there for you to figure out. Use your common sense to interpret anything that isn't clear.

Answer Choice Strategies

☑ Answer Selection

The most thorough way to pick an answer choice is to identify and eliminate wrong answers until only one is left, then confirm it is the correct answer. Sometimes an answer choice may immediately seem right, but be careful. The test writers will usually put more than one reasonable answer choice on each question, so take a second to read all of them and make sure that the other choices are not equally obvious. As long as you have time left, it is better to read every answer choice than to pick the first one that looks right without checking the others.

☑ Answer Choice Families

An answer choice family consists of two (in rare cases, three) answer choices that are very similar in construction and cannot all be true at the same time. If you see two answer choices that are direct opposites or parallels, one of them is usually the correct answer. For instance, if one answer choice says that quantity x increases and another either says that quantity x decreases (opposite) or says that quantity y increases (parallel), then those answer choices would fall into the same family. An answer choice that doesn't match the construction of the answer choice family is more likely to be incorrect. Most questions will not have answer choice families, but when they do appear, you should be prepared to recognize them.

☑ Eliminate Answers

Eliminate answer choices as soon as you realize they are wrong, but make sure you consider all possibilities. If you are eliminating answer choices and realize that the last one you are left with is also wrong, don't panic. Start over and consider each choice again. There may be something you missed the first time that you will realize on the second pass.

☑ Avoid Fact Traps

Don't be distracted by an answer choice that is factually true but doesn't answer the question. You are looking for the choice that answers the question. Stay focused on what the question is asking for so you don't accidentally pick an answer that is true but incorrect. Always go back to the question and make sure the answer choice you've selected actually answers the question and is not merely a true statement.

☑ Extreme Statements

In general, you should avoid answers that put forth extreme actions as standard practice or proclaim controversial ideas as established fact. An answer choice that states the "process should be used in certain situations, if..." is much more likely to be correct than one that states the "process should be discontinued completely." The first is a calm rational statement and doesn't even make a definitive, uncompromising stance, using a hedge word *if* to provide wiggle room, whereas the second choice is far more extreme.

⊘ Benchmark

As you read through the answer choices and you come across one that seems to answer the question well, mentally select that answer choice. This is not your final answer, but it's the one that will help you evaluate the other answer choices. The one that you selected is your benchmark or standard for judging each of the other answer choices. Every other answer choice must be compared to your benchmark. That choice is correct until proven otherwise by another answer choice beating it. If you find a better answer, then that one becomes your new benchmark. Once you've decided that no other choice answers the question as well as your benchmark, you have your final answer.

⊘ Predict the Answer

Before you even start looking at the answer choices, it is often best to try to predict the answer. When you come up with the answer on your own, it is easier to avoid distractions and traps because you will know exactly what to look for. The right answer choice is unlikely to be word-for-word what you came up with, but it should be a close match. Even if you are confident that you have the right answer, you should still take the time to read each option before moving on.

General Strategies

⊘ Tough Questions

If you are stumped on a problem or it appears too hard or too difficult, don't waste time. Move on! Remember though, if you can quickly check for obviously incorrect answer choices, your chances of guessing correctly are greatly improved. Before you completely give up, at least try to knock out a couple of possible answers. Eliminate what you can and then guess at the remaining answer choices before moving on.

⊘ Check Your Work

Since you will probably not know every term listed and the answer to every question, it is important that you get credit for the ones that you do know. Don't miss any questions through careless mistakes. If at all possible, try to take a second to look back over your answer selection and make sure you've selected the correct answer choice and haven't made a costly careless mistake (such as marking an answer choice that you didn't mean to mark). This quick double check should more than pay for itself in caught mistakes for the time it costs.

⊘ Pace Yourself

It's easy to be overwhelmed when you're looking at a page full of questions; your mind is confused and full of random thoughts, and the clock is ticking down faster than you would like. Calm down and maintain the pace that you have set for yourself. Especially as you get down to the last few minutes of the test, don't let the small numbers on the clock make you panic. As long as you are on track by monitoring your pace, you are guaranteed to have time for each question.

⊘ Don't Rush

It is very easy to make errors when you are in a hurry. Maintaining a fast pace in answering questions is pointless if it makes you miss questions that you would have gotten right otherwise. Test writers like to include distracting information and wrong answers that seem right. Taking a little extra time to avoid careless mistakes can make all the difference in your test score. Find a pace that allows you to be confident in the answers that you select.

⊘ Keep Moving

Panicking will not help you pass the test, so do your best to stay calm and keep moving. Taking deep breaths and going through the answer elimination steps you practiced can help to break through a stress barrier and keep your pace.

Final Notes

The combination of a solid foundation of content knowledge and the confidence that comes from practicing your plan for applying that knowledge is the key to maximizing your performance on test day. As your foundation of content knowledge is built up and strengthened, you'll find that the strategies included in this chapter become more and more effective in helping you quickly sift through the distractions and traps of the test to isolate the correct answer.

Now that you're preparing to move forward into the test content chapters of this book, be sure to keep your goal in mind. As you read, think about how you will be able to apply this information on the test. If you've already seen sample questions for the test and you have an idea of the question format and style, try to come up with questions of your own that you can answer based on what you're reading. This will give you valuable practice applying your knowledge in the same ways you can expect to on test day.

Good luck and good studying!

Esophagus

Esophageal Anatomy

The esophagus is muscular and about 25 cm long. The esophagus has two sphincters. The upper esophageal sphincter is made up of striated muscle and acts like a valve to prohibit air from getting into the GI tract. The lower esophageal sphincter is made up of smooth muscle and has a baseline muscle tone to prohibit the reflux of acid into the esophagus. The proximal esophagus is composed of striated muscle, and the distal esophagus has smooth muscle. The middle esophagus transitions from striated muscle to smooth muscle. The musculature is oriented in an inner circular layer and a longitudinal layer.

Peristalsis

Peristalsis is defined as "a sequential coordinated contraction wave that travels the entire length of the esophagus, propelling intraluminal contents distally to the stomach." The lower esophageal sphincter relaxes upon swallowing and stays open until the wave of peristalsis ventures through the sphincter, at which point the lower esophageal sphincter closes. Primary peristalsis is stimulated upon swallowing; this peristaltic wave has a speed of 2 cm/s. Secondary peristalsis occurs due to esophageal distention and functions to rid the esophagus of residual food or of reflux. Tertiary contractions are not peristaltic and are considered dysfunctional.

Disorders of Esophageal Motility

Esophageal motility disorders are relatively common and include primary disorders and secondary disorders. Secondary disorders are often due to a systemic disease process. The clinical presentation of an esophageal motility disorder may be varied, but 80% of patients have dysphagia and chest pain. Examples of esophageal motility disorders include achalasia, diffuse esophageal spasm, nutcracker esophagus, hypertensive lower esophageal sphincter, inefficient esophageal motility disorder, and secondary motility disorders (scleroderma, diabetes, alcoholism, psychiatric disorders, and presbyesophagus). Achalasia is the best-understood disorder of esophageal motility and is the only disorder with well-defined pathology.

Achalasia

Achalasia is a disorder of esophageal motility that involves the loss of ganglion cells from the esophageal wall. The loss of ganglion cells starts at the lower esophageal sphincter and then travels proximally. Pathology involved in achalasia is a result of the lack of inhibitory nerves at the lower esophageal sphincter (LES), which leads to an inability of the LES to relax that result in obstruction. The lack of ganglion cells along the body of the esophagus contributes to a lack of peristalsis that yields food stasis and esophageal distention. Botulinum toxin injections may help relax the LES.

Gastroesophageal Reflux Disease (GERD)

There are numerous factors in the etiology of gastroesophageal reflux disease (GERD). Factors implicated include disorders of motility, damage, resistance, and others. Motility disorders that contribute to GERD include intermittent lower esophageal relaxation, ineffective lower esophageal sphincter, ineffective esophageal peristalsis, scleroderma, CREST syndrome, and delayed gastric emptying. Damage factors include elevated gastric acid production, bile, and pancreatic juices. Resistance factors include decreased saliva and bicarbonate production, decreased mucosal blood flow, and growth factors/protective mucus. Other factors may include obesity, hiatal hernia, and possibly obstructive sleep apnea.

GERD is defined as "chronic symptoms of heartburn, acid regurgitation or dysfunction, or injury to the esophagus or other organs because of abnormal reflux of gastric contents." In the United States, 18% of adults have symptoms of GERD every week; 40% have GERD symptoms every month. GERD symptoms are more likely with increasing age and are rare in Chinese, Japanese, and other Asians. Upon endoscopy, 10% of patients have benign strictures, 4% have Barrett's esophagus, and only a very small number of patients have adenocarcinoma.

Review Video: Peptic Ulcers and GERD
Visit mometrix.com/academy and enter code: 184332

Review Video: GERD
Visit mometrix.com/academy and enter code: 294757

Gastric Factors

GERD may be a result of gastric factors such as delayed gastric emptying or elevated gastric acid. GERD may be seen in patients with Zollinger-Ellison syndrome, patients in a reclining position, or patients with abdominal straining. The right lateral decubitus position is associated with increased episodes of GERD. If reflux occurs after the stomach contents have been maximally buffered (usually in the first hour after ingestion of food), and at maximal stomach distention, the reflux is not as severe because of the elevated pH of the gastric contents

Helicobacter Pylori

A popular treatment of active duodenal ulcers was the eradication of *Helicobacter pylori*. Some data show that getting rid of *Helicobacter pylori* in the treatment of a duodenal ulcer may increase the risk of GERD, because chronic infection with *H. pylori* may be a protective mechanism against GERD. Research shows that chronic infection or poorly eradicated *H. pylori* may result in chronic atrophic gastritis in the stomach, which may diminish acid production and thus be a protective device against GERD. Some studies suggest that heightened GERD symptoms after elimination of *H. pylori* could be a result of increased acid production.

Esophageal Symptoms

Esophageal symptoms of GERD include heartburn and regurgitation of acid. Often, patients describe a decrease in symptoms with the ingestion of antacids or the ingestion of milk. Other esophageal symptoms associated with GERD may include hyper-salivation (water brash), trouble swallowing (dysphagia), swallowing that is painful (odynophagia), and chest pain. Symptoms of GERD may happen at any time but are much more common within 1 to 3 hours after ingesting a meal. GERD is thought to be the most common cause of non-cardiac chest pain. Esophageal chest pain may be hard to differentiate initially from cardiac chest pain.

Lower Esophageal Sphincter

The lower esophageal sphincter serves as a barrier to the reflux of gastric material into the esophagus. The components of the lower esophageal sphincter and its attachments include the smooth muscle of the lower esophageal sphincter, gastric sling fibers, and the striated muscle of the crural diaphragm. The lower esophageal sphincter maintains its tone when at rest and relaxes when swallowing and gastric distention occurs. This is also known as a venting reflex. In the presence of GERD, the resting tone of the lower esophageal sphincter is breached easily and allows reflux of gastric contents into the esophagus.

Mechanism of Acid Clearance

The mechanism of acid clearance from the esophagus is due to gravity and peristalsis, which are thought to be volume clearance factors, and due to the buffering factors provided by the saliva and by bicarbonate. Saliva and bicarbonate serve to buffer the mucosa and are considered chemical neutralization mechanisms. In some patients with GERD, acid clearance is impaired due to ineffective peristalsis or due to ineffective buffering from saliva or bicarbonate. Ineffective peristalsis may be a result of a connective tissue disease such as scleroderma or due to the CREST syndrome.

Extra-Esophageal Symptoms

Some of the extra-esophageal symptoms of GERD may include chronic cough, chronic wheezing, sore throat, persistent hoarseness, chronic post-nasal drip, frequent clearing of the throat, neck pain, throat pain, trouble swallowing, apnea, and earache. GERD is postulated to produce extra-esophageal symptoms by either direct aggravation of the larynx, trachea, or bronchial structures, or by functional changes that are caused by reflex. In order to attribute extra-esophageal symptoms to GERD, diagnostic measures need to be undertaken or empiric treatment with acid-blocking medications needs to be utilized in order to rule out other potential causes.

Diagnostic Measures

Most patients with GERD do not require diagnostic testing, since the first step is usually an empiric trial of acid-suppressing medications. Diagnostic measures are indicated, however, in patients with alarming or atypical symptoms or patients with lackluster results to an empiric medication trial. Diagnostic tests may include endoscopy, contrast radiography, 24-hour ambulatory pH testing, Bernstein testing, or gastroesophageal scintigraphy. Endoscopy serves to allow direct visualization of the esophagus, to identify reflux esophagitis, to perform biopsies of Barrett's and adenocarcinoma, and to dilate strictures, whereas contrast studies are useful in identifying hiatal hernia.

Treatment

The treatment of GERD includes lifestyle changes, neutralization of acid, suppression of acid, prokinetics, and mechanical reflux prevention. Lifestyle changes include elevating the head of the bed, not ingesting food within 3 hours of bed, eating smaller-sized meals with less fat content, decreasing ingestion of caffeine and chocolate, and quitting smoking. Neutralization of acid involves the use of antacids, chewing gum, and alginate compounds. Suppression of acid involves the utilization of H-2 blocking agents and proton-pump inhibiting agents. Metoclopramide is a prokinetic medication that has been used in the treatment of GERD. Mechanical reflux prevention includes lap surgery and endoscopic treatments.

Barrett's Esophagus

Barrett's esophagus is a condition in which cell metaplasia occurs in the inferior aspect of the esophagus. The lower esophagus is normally composed of squamous epithelium; however, in the presence of Barrett's esophagus, the squamous epithelium is replaced by metaplastic goblet and columnar cells. Barrett's esophagus is strongly linked to adenocarcinoma of the esophagus. Barrett's esophagus is thought to be the result of chronic exposure to gastric acid and is linked to GERD; it occurs in 5 to 15% of patients with GERD and is classified as a pre-malignant condition.

Symptoms

The symptoms of Barrett's esophagus may include recurrent and chronic heartburn, difficulty swallowing (dysphagia), hematemesis, pain under the sternum at the junction of the esophagus and the stomach, and unexplained weight loss that is thought to be a result of eating being too painful.

The risk of Barrett's esophagus has been shown to be greater in those with central obesity. The normal population has a prevalence of Barrett's esophagus of 1.6%. The incidence of Barrett's esophagus in the United States is thought to be 8 times higher in white men than in white women.

Diagnosis

Barrett's esophagus is typically diagnosed via EGD (esophagogastroduodenoscopy) and biopsy. The cells that are frequently associated with Barrett's esophagus on biopsy are characterized in four categories: non-dysplastic, low-grade dysplasia, high-grade dysplasia, and frank carcinoma. It is recommended that patients with non-dysplastic cells or with low-grade dysplasia have an annual EGD. Patients with high-grade dysplasia or frank carcinoma are typically advised to undergo surgery. With high-grade dysplasia, the risk of adenocarcinoma of the esophagus is estimated to be 10% per patient-year or possibly even higher. Adenocarcinoma of the esophagus has a very high mortality.

Treatment

The initial treatment of Barrett's esophagus is to treat acid reflux in order to prevent or to slow the development of changes associated with the condition. There are numerous treatments that specifically focus upon Barrett's esophagus. One such targeted treatment is that of photodynamic therapy (PDT) wherein a laser is used via an endoscope to ablate abnormal cells in the esophagus after pre-treatment with porfimer sodium, which causes such cells to be light-sensitive. Another treatment is endoscopic mucosal resection (EMR) in which the abnormal mucosal lining is resected from the esophageal wall. Finally, surgery may be used to resect a large portion of the esophagus.

Esophageal Cancer

Cancer of the esophagus is usually either adenocarcinoma or squamous cell carcinoma. Adenocarcinoma of the esophagus is more common in the last 20 years than squamous cell carcinoma of the esophagus, and has been thought to account for 50% of new cases of cancer of the esophagus. In the 1970s, squamous cell carcinoma of the esophagus caused 90-95% of all cases of cancer of the esophagus and primarily was found in black men with a long history of tobacco and ethanol use. Adenocarcinoma primarily occurs in white men and is associated with GERD and the development of Barrett's esophagus.

Risk Factors

Esophageal cancer is thought to be a result of repeated exposure of the lining of the esophagus to noxious stimuli. In the Chinese, esophageal cancer is thought to be a result of vitamin and nutritional deficiencies (especially riboflavin deficiency). Wu and associates did a genome-wide association study, which served to identify loci on certain chromosomes that implicate multiple gene loci, interaction between such genes, and the environment in the development of esophageal cancer. In western society, the most common risk factors for squamous cell carcinoma are cigarette smoking and alcohol use. GERD is the most common risk factor for adenocarcinoma.

Symptoms

The most common symptom in the clinical presentation of cancer of the esophagus is dysphagia; the dysphagia starts with solids but soon progresses to liquids. Weight loss is the next most common finding in the clinical presentation of cancer of the esophagus. Half of patients with esophageal cancer have weight loss, and some have bleeding. Pain is typically located in the epigastric region or in the retrosternal area. The presence of hoarseness usually indicates involvement of the recurrent laryngeal nerve and is considered evidence of unresectability. Chronic and persistent cough may also be present.

Laboratory Tests

Laboratory tests, such as BUN, creatinine, albumin, and liver function tests need to be obtained to assess the nutritional status in light of dysphagia and to assess liver function. Imaging studies can include a barium swallow to identify the anatomy of the distal esophagus if endoscopy cannot be performed. EGD enables direct visualization of the tumor and biopsy of the tumor. Endoscopic ultrasound is thought to be the most sensitive means by which to assess the penetration depth of the tumor and to assess for peri-esophageal node involvement. CT scans of the chest and abdomen are used to identify metastases to the lungs or the liver.

Classifications

TMN classification of cancer of the esophagus is as follows:

- Tis-carcinoma in situ/high-grade dysplasia
- T1-Lamina propria or submucosa
- T1a-Lamina propria or muscularis mucosae
- T1b-Submucosa
- T2-Muscularis propria
- T3-Adventitia
- T4-Adjacent structures
- T4a-Pleura, pericardium, diaphragm, or adjacent peritoneum
- T4b-Other adjacent structures (e. G. aorta, vertebral body, trachea)
- NO-No regional lymph node metastasis
- N1- 1-2 regional lymph nodes (N1 is site-dependent)
- N2- 3-6 regional lymph nodes
- N3- More than six regional lymph nodes
- M1- Distant metastasis (M1a and M1b are site-dependent)

All esophageal tumors and tumors with epicenters within 5 cm of the esophagogastric junction that also extend into the esophagus are classified and staged according to the esophageal scheme.

Medical Management

Typically, medical management of esophageal cancer is utilized for patients that are not surgical candidates because of clinical diseases or the presence of advanced disease. The primary goal of medical management is to help with dysphagia and to facilitate eating. Chemotherapy as a mono-modality in the treatment of cancer of the esophagus is very limited, whereas radiation alone will improve dysphagia in 50% of patients. Chemotherapy combined with radiation therapy has been used with success as a pre-operative adjunct in patients with advanced esophageal cancer. Laser treatment may give relief of dysphagia in 70% of patients.

Surgical Management

Surgical treatment is a vital aspect of the management of cancer of the esophagus. Esophagectomy can be accomplished either by performing abdominal and cervical incisions utilizing blunt dissection of the mediastinum via the esophageal hiatus (transhiatal esophagectomy) or by performing abdominal and right thoracic incisions (transthoracic esophagectomy). The transhiatal esophagectomy has the advantages of not having a chest incision that may lengthen recovery time and that may compromise lung function. In this procedure, the continuity of the GI tract can be reestablished utilizing the stomach. This procedure, however, does not give direct visualization and not as many lymph nodes can be resected.

Esophagitis

Esophagitis in HIV infection typically results in odynophagia and dysphagia. The cause is usually a *Candida* infection or may also be secondary to CMV, herpes simplex, nonspecific ulcerations, and MAC. Kaposi sarcoma, lymphoma, and GERD may also be factors. The CD4 count is helpful in formulating the diagnostic evaluation of esophagitis in HIV infection. For example, patients with esophagitis due to *Candida* and herpes simplex are most likely to have a CD4 count of less than 200. CMV and nonspecific ulcerations are only seen in patients with a CD4 count of less than 100.

Symptoms of odynophagia and dysphagia are not diagnostic as to the causes of esophagitis in HIV infection and require work-up. Barium swallow may exhibit findings that may indicate neoplasm or infection; however, endoscopy with biopsy is considered the optimum means to establish a diagnostic cause of odynophagia and dysphagia. During endoscopy and biopsy, the mucosa in its entirety must be examined. Areas that suggest *Candida* infection must be scraped in order to check the underlying tissue for any pathologic findings. The presence of ulcers requires more than 6 biopsies in order to determine etiology.

Most clinicians utilize empiric therapy to manage the symptoms of odynophagia and dysphagia in esophagitis of HIV infection. The most likely cause of symptoms of esophagitis in HIV infection is *Candida* infection. Empiric treatment with fluconazole or itraconazole is often utilized because they have been demonstrated to be more effective than ketoconazole. The main treatment goal is to decrease or eliminate the symptoms of odynophagia and dysphagia in order to maximize nutritional intake. Amphotericin B is used in the treatment of refractory candida infections. Nonspecific ulcers typically need treatment with steroids.

GI Symptoms of Sjögren Syndrome

The GI symptoms of Sjögren syndrome are numerous and are primarily due to lack of secretions. Over dryness of the pharynx and the esophagus results in problems swallowing and food getting "stuck" in the throat. The lack of saliva results in an impaired acid clearance that can lead to GERD and esophagitis. Patients may experience pain in the abdomen and diarrhea. Some patients develop acute or chronic pancreatitis with malabsorption from pancreatic insufficiency. Patients with Sjögren syndrome also exhibit symptoms of delayed gastric emptying which may include early satiety, abdominal pain, nausea, and vomiting.

GI Manifestations of Systemic Mastocytosis

Systemic mastocytosis is classified as a myeloproliferative neoplasm and signs and symptoms are secondary to the accumulation of mast cells in the bone marrow, spleen, skin, liver, and the GI tract. Involvement of the GI tract is characterized by mast cell infiltration in the liver, pancreas, and intestines. GI tract issues in systemic mastocytosis include esophagitis, esophageal stricture, esophageal varices, peptic ulcer disease, dilated small intestine, malabsorption, multiple polyposis, diverticulitis, hepatomegaly, portal hypertension, ascites, sclerosing cholangitis, and Budd-Chiari syndrome. The most common GI symptoms of systemic mastocytosis are abdominal pain, nausea, vomiting, and diarrhea.

GI Manifestations of Diabetes

GI symptoms of diabetes may be numerous and may involve the entire GI tract from the mouth to the anus. Studies show that 75% of patients in diabetic clinics will have GI symptoms. Common symptoms include dysphagia, early satiety, GERD, constipation, abdominal pain, nausea, vomiting, and diarrhea. Poor glycemic control is linked to a higher incidence of GI problems. Other GI conditions that may be seen in patients with diabetes are gastroparesis, ulcers, *Candida* infections, small bowel motility issues, malabsorption, bacterial overgrowth syndrome, diarrhea, and pancreatic exocrine disorders resulting in problems digesting fats, carbohydrates, and proteins.

Skin Findings That Indicate Esophageal Disease

Plummer-Vinson syndrome is characterized by chronic dysphagia, iron deficiency, and esophageal webs. Skin findings in Plummer-Vinson include koilonychias, loss of teeth, cheilosis, tongue atrophy, and stomatitis. Dystrophic epidermolysis bullosa may have concomitant esophageal strictures that are due to trauma from repeated food ingestion as well as esophageal web development, constipation, and anal stenosis. 90% of patients with scleroderma have GI manifestations that are a result of excess collagen production, overactive immune system response, and impaired cellular immune response. GI symptoms of scleroderma include fullness, reflux esophagitis, dysphagia, and abdominal pain.

Stomach/Duodenum

Peptic Ulcer Disease

The most typical symptom of peptic ulcer disease is epigastric pain that is described as gnawing or burning and that usually happens right after eating. It is important to test for *H. pylori* in patients with peptic ulcers and to treat appropriately. An upper GI endoscopy is usually used as a diagnostic measure for peptic ulcer disease because it allows direct visualization of the ulcer, assessment of any bleeding, and a means for hemostasis if indicated. The treatment for *H. pylori* infection is proton pump inhibitor (PPI)-based triple therapy, which typically results in ulcer healing in 85-90% of patients.

Peptic ulcers are "defects in the gastric or duodenal mucosa that extend through the muscularis mucosa." Peptic ulcers occur as a result of disruption of the normal balance between acid production and mucus protective production. Factors that contribute to injury include nonsteroidal antiinflammatory use, *H. pylori* infection, alcohol use, bile salts, acid, and pepsin; such factors can let hydrogen ions diffuse in a reverse fashion, which can cause injury to the epithelial cells. *H. pylori* infection was initially found to be a mechanism in peptic ulcer disease in 1983 and is a part of a triad that also includes acid and pepsin.

Etiology

The following factors have been implicated in the etiology of peptic ulcer disease: *H. pylori* infection, drugs, lifestyle, severe physiologic stress, hypersecretory states, and genetic issues. The two most common factors in peptic ulcer disease are *H. pylori* infection and the use of nonsteroidal anti-inflammatory drugs (NSAIDs). NSAIDs disrupt the mucosal barrier, which allows injury. The following factors contribute to an elevated risk of peptic ulcer disease with NSAID use: previous peptic ulcer, older age, female gender, high doses, combined medications, anticoagulant administration, and comorbid illnesses. Tobacco and alcohol use have been also implicated in peptic ulcer disease.

Conditions that contribute to severe physiologic stress, such as burns, trauma to the CNS, surgery, critical illness, sepsis, hypotension, respiratory failure, and multi-system trauma, can cause peptic ulcers. Cushing ulcers are deep ulcers that have a high rate of perforation and are typically found with brain tumors/injury; Curling ulcers are frequently seen with severe burn injuries. It is rare for hypersecretory states to cause peptic ulcers; however, the following states can contribute: Zollinger-Ellison syndrome, MEN-1, antral G-cell hyperplasia, systemic mastocytosis, basophilic leukemias, cystic fibrosis, short bowel syndrome, and hyperparathyroidism. Approximately 20% of patients with duodenal ulcers have a positive family history.

Associated Factors

The following factors have been associated with peptic ulcer disease: cirrhosis; chronic obstructive pulmonary disease; allergic gastritis; eosinophilic gastritis; CMV infection; graft versus host disease; gastropathy of uremia; Henoch-Schönlein gastritis; corrosive gastropathy; celiac disease; bile gastropathy; autoimmune disease; Crohn disease; sarcoidosis; tuberculosis; histiocytosis X; phlegmonous gastritis ; emphysematous gastritis; infections such as Epstein-Barr, HIV, *H. heilmannii*, herpes simplex, influenza, syphilis, *Candida*, histoplasmosis, mucormycosis, and anisakiasis; chemotherapy agents (5-fluorouracil, methotrexate, and cyclophosphamide); local radiation; and crack-cocaine use (which contributes to intense vasoconstriction, decreased blood flow, which, in turn, leads to mucosal damage).

Symptoms

The most commonly encountered symptom of peptic ulcer disease is epigastric pain. Duodenal ulcer pain typically occurs 2 to 3 hours after eating and often wakes the patient up at night. Other symptoms may include the following: dyspepsia, heartburn, chest pain, melena or hematemesis, hematochezia, and fatigue/dyspnea (symptoms of anemia). Sudden symptom occurrence may indicate perforation. Alarming symptoms include bleeding, anemia, unintentional and unexplained weight loss, early satiety, dysphagia/odynophagia that is progressive in nature, frequent and recurrent emesis, and a positive family history of gastrointestinal malignancy. A guaiac-positive stool may indicate occult blood loss on physical examination.

Laboratory Tests

Laboratory tests, such as CBC, liver function, amylase, and lipase may be needed as well as testing for *H. pylori* (rapid urease test, histopathology, culture). Upper GI endoscopy is the usual diagnostic tool to detect peptic ulcer disease; it is highly sensitive and allows for biopsy. Gastric ulcers typically are solitary lesions with a "punched-out smooth ulcer base" and often are located at the junction between the fundus and the antrum. Benign peptic ulcers are usually smooth in appearance, whereas malignant peptic ulcers are irregular in appearance, with nodular folds around the ulcer.

Differential Diagnosis

Numerous conditions may be included in the differential diagnosis of peptic ulcer disease. Such conditions include acute coronary syndrome, functional dyspepsia, Zollinger-Ellison syndrome, Crohn disease, abdominal aortic aneurysm, cholangitis, cholecystitis, cholelithiasis, diverticular disease, perforation of the esophagus, tears of the esophagus, esophageal rupture, acute and chronic gastritis, gastroenteritis, gastroesophageal reflux disease, inflammatory bowel disease, and viral hepatitis. The diagnosis of functional dyspepsia or non-ulcer dyspepsia is thought to be one of exclusion, because these patients have long-standing epigastric pain with no findings on diagnostic evaluation.

Treatment

The treatment choices for peptic ulcer disease include empiric anti-secretory medications, empiric triple therapy for *H. pylori* infection, initial upper GI endoscopy with appropriate therapeutic measures, and definitive *H. pylori* treatment for documented infection. Upper GI endoscopy is necessary to rule out gastric carcinoma and to document healing of gastric ulcers; endoscopy is typically undertaken 6 to 8 weeks after initial diagnosis. Indications for surgery in the treatment of peptic ulcer disease include failure of endoscopic hemostasis, recurrent bleeding despite endoscopic hemostasis, and perforation. Techniques may include oversewing of the ulcer, vagotomy, pyloroplasty, Billroth I, Billroth II, and highly selective vagotomy.

Prognosis

If the cause of peptic ulcer disease is addressed, an excellent prognosis is expected. Many patients have treatment of *H. pylori* infections, not using NSAID medications, and the use of antisecretory medications. Successful treatment of *H. pylori* infection decreases the recurrence rate of ulcers from 60-90% to 10-20%. Perforation incidence of NSAID-induced ulcers is about 0.3% per patient year while the incidence of obstruction is 0.1% per patient year. Mortality for peptic ulcer disease is one death per 100,000. Mortality rate for ulcer hemorrhage is around 5%.

Gastritis

Gastritis is considered an irritation or inflammation of the stomach lining and is characterized by symptoms of dyspepsia. Gastritis may be an acute condition or may be a chronic condition. Gastritis is common; 10% of patients presenting to emergency departments have symptoms of gastritis. Causes of gastritis may include the following medications, medical and surgical conditions, stressors, lifestyle habits, chemicals, and various infections. Symptoms of gastritis may include upper abdominal pain, belching, nausea and vomiting, and bloating. Pain associated with gastritis is frequently described as sharp, stabbing, or gnawing.

Causes

Many medications are known to causes gastritis and include aspirin and aspirin derivatives, nonsteroidal anti-inflammatory drugs, steroids, potassium supplements, iron supplements, and chemotherapeutic medications. The ingestion of chemicals such as lye or acid ingestion may cause gastritis, as may the ingestion of foreign bodies such as paper clips or pins. Various medical and surgical conditions may cause gastritis; for example, critical medical illness or injury, medical procedures (e.g., endoscopy), post-gastrectomy, radiation treatment, autoimmune diseases, pernicious anemia, and protracted vomiting. Infections like tuberculosis, syphilis, viruses, bacteria, fungal, and parasites also may cause gastritis.

Diagnostic Tests

Certain tests may be ordered and include *H. pylori*, CBC, liver and renal function, UA, gallbladder and pancreas screens, HCG, and stool testing for occult blood. Endoscopy may be indicated for visualization of the stomach lining and for obtaining biopsy. Plain x-rays yield little in the diagnosis of gastritis. An upper GI series with barium swallow is sometimes used to demonstrate erosions or ulcers in the lining of the stomach. Upper GI endoscopy, however, is more sensitive as a diagnostic tool for gastritis since it allows for actual visualization of the lining of the stomach and for biopsy.

Treatment

There are numerous treatment options for gastritis. Antacids are frequently employed and may include the brands Maalox, Alka Seltzer, and Rolaids. Such medications work by neutralizing stomach acid. H_2 blocking agents (including brands such as Pepcid, Zantac, and Tagamet) may be utilized to decrease the symptoms of gastritis by lowering acid production. Proton pump inhibitors (PPI) are medications (omeprazole, omeprazole/sodium bicarbonate, lansoprazole, pantoprazole, and rabeprazole) that function to lower acid production and are often more efficacious than the H_2 blockers. It is important to test for and to treat the presence of *H. pylori*, typically with amoxicillin and clarithromycin.

Gastric Cancer

Gastric cancer is the 14th most common cancer in the United States and is the 2nd most common cause of cancer-related death in the world. The decrease in the incidence of gastric cancer has been attributed to refrigeration, increased fruit and vegetable consumption, lower salt intake, and decreased food contamination. Another aspect potentially related to the decline in the incidence of gastric cancer is the increased screening for and treatment of chronic *H. pylori* infection. Gastric cancer is typically quite difficult to treat and cure, because most patients present with an advanced form of the disease.

Pathophysiology

Gastric cancer is typically classified based upon its location in relation to the long axis of the stomach. 40% of gastric cancer occurs in the lower aspect of the stomach, 40% occurs in the mid-portion, and 15% occurs in the upper aspect, with 10% occurring in more than one location of the stomach. The decline in the incidence and the mortality of gastric cancer in the United States has been mainly in gastric cancers located in the lower aspect of the stomach, whereas the incidence of adenocarcinoma in the cardia is increasing.

Epidemiology

Gastric cancer is the 7th leading cause of cancer-related death in the United States, the 4th most common cause of cancer in the world, and the 2nd most common cause of cancer-related death in the world. The incidence of gastric cancer is highest in Asia and certain areas of South America, and lowest in the United States. The highest death rates from gastric cancer are found in Chile, Japan, South America, and Russia. In the United States, the highest incidence of gastric cancer occurs in those of Asian and Pacific Islander ethnicity.

Clinical Presentation

In the United States, 25% of patients with gastric cancer have localized disease, 31% have regional disease, and 32% show metastatic disease. The early symptoms of gastric cancer may be vague, and most patients typically present with symptoms that reflect advanced cancer, such as indigestion, nausea, vomiting, dysphagia, postprandial fullness or bloating, anorexia, melena, hematemesis, and weight loss. Advanced disease may exhibit malignant peritoneal and pleural effusions, gastric outlet obstruction, gastric bleeding secondary to esophageal varices, jaundice (intrahepatic or extrahepatic), cachexia, and signs of starvation. Most physical findings are indicators of advanced disease.

Causes

Dietary causes of gastric cancer include large amounts of pickled vegetables, salted fish, and smoked meats. Diets high in foods with vitamin C, such as fruits and fresh vegetables, appear to have a protective effect. Smoking is linked to gastric cancer and is dose- and duration-dependent; smoking increases the risk of gastric cancer 1.6 fold, especially in men. *H. pylori* infection has a strong association with the development of gastric cancer due to chronic atrophic gastritis and increases the risk 6 fold. Most gastric cancers due to *H. pylori* are located in the antrum, body, and fundus.

Having had a previous gastric surgery is a risk factor for gastric cancer, possibly as a result of altered stomach pH. Gastric polyps have also been implicated as a risk factor for gastric cancer. 10% of patients with gastric cancer have a positive family history; certain hereditary conditions are also associated with gastric cancer, such as hereditary non-polyposis colorectal cancer, Li-Fraumeni syndrome, familial adenomatous polyposis, and Peutz-Jeghers syndrome. Other possible causes of gastric cancer include Epstein-Barr virus (lymphoepithelioma-like carcinoma), pernicious anemia (due to advanced atrophic gastritis), obesity, radiation exposure, and possible oral bisphosphonates.

Diagnosis, Testing, and Imaging

The differential diagnosis for gastric cancer includes esophageal cancer, esophageal stricture, esophagitis, gastric ulcer, acute gastritis, atrophic gastritis, chronic gastritis, bacterial gastroenteritis, viral gastroenteritis, non-Hodgkin's lymphoma, and cancers of the small intestine. Laboratory tests that may be used in the diagnosis of gastric cancer include CBC (30% of patients with gastric cancer are anemic); electrolyte panel; liver function tests; carcinoembryonic antigen (CEA), which is elevated in 45-50% of patients with gastric cancer; and cancer antigen 19-9 (CA), which is elevated in approximately 20% of patients diagnosed with gastric cancer. Obtaining laboratory studies also aids in selecting the optimum treatment.

EGD has been shown to have a diagnostic accuracy of 95% and facilitates biopsy of the lesion for tissue diagnosis. Any ulcerated lesion needs to have at least 6 different specimens obtained due to the possibility of variable states of malignant transformation. The use of endoscopic ultrasound can be helpful in assessing the penetration depth of the tumor and in assessing for involvement of adjacent structures. If unable to perform upper GI endoscopy, double-contrast upper-GI series and barium swallow can be used, but is considered only 75% accurate.

Histology

95% of gastric cancer is caused by adenocarcinoma, and lymphomas are the second most common type of gastric cancer. 2% of gastric cancer is of stromal origin (leiomyoma or leiomyosarcoma) and 1% of gastric cancer is carcinoid. Adenoacanthoma and squamous cell each account for 1%. Adenocarcinoma is further classified by the following descriptive histology: tubular, papillary, mucinous, signet-ring cells, and undifferentiated. Gross appearance of the tumor may also be used for classification; such descriptions include ulcerative, polypoid, scirrhous (diffuse linitis plastica), superficial spreading, multicentric, or Barrett ectopic adenocarcinoma.

TMN Staging

Primary tumor: TX—primary tumor unable to be assessed; T0—no evidence of primary tumor; Tis—carcinoma-in-situ, intraepithelial tumor without invasion of lamina propria; T1—invades lamina propria or submucosa; T2—invades muscularis propria or subserosa; T3—invades serosa without adjacent structures; and T4—invades adjacent structures. Regional lymph nodes: NX—nodes can't be assessed; N0—no regional lymph node metastasis; N1—metastasis in 1-6 nodes; N2—metastasis in 7-15 regional lymph nodes; and N3—metastasis in more than 15 regional lymph nodes. Distant metastasis: MX—distant metastasis is unable to be assessed; M0—no distant metastasis identified; M1—distant metastasis is identified. (American Joint Committee on Cancer Staging Manual, 2006.)

Prognosis and Spread Pattern

The prognosis of gastric cancer is highly influenced by the depth of the tumor into the wall of the stomach and the presence or the absence of regional lymph node involvement. A dire prognosis is associated with linitis plastica (large area of the wall of the stomach or the entire stomach with extensive infiltration); this is typically found in 5% of patients with gastric cancer. Positive tumor margins and the presence of regional lymph nodes also portend a poor prognosis. The spread pattern of gastric cancer may be direct, lymphatic, or hematogenous.

Surgical Treatment

In the United States, the following surgical procedures are performed for the treatment of gastric cancer: total gastrectomy, esophagogastrectomy (for tumors of the cardia and gastroesophageal junction), and sub-total gastrectomy (for tumors of the distal aspect of the stomach). There is an extensive network of lymphatics surrounding the stomach; therefore, it has been customary to obtain a 5 cm margin both proximally and distally to the tumor. Aggressive lymph node dissection is generally recommended, with the D2 dissection preferred as suggested by the National Comprehensive Cancer Network. D2 dissection involves node dissection of the following areas: hepatic left gastric, celiac, and splenic arteries, and arteries in the splenic hilum.

Gastric Motility Disorders

Gastric motility disorders are somewhat common. Examples of such disorders include gastroparesis (delayed gastric emptying), dumping syndrome (rapid gastric emptying), and functional dyspepsia. Gastroparesis may be simply idiopathic or may be caused by the pylorus and duodenum being blocked by an ulcer or by a tumor, the pylorus and duodenum being obstructed by large or indigestible material, the pyloric sphincter malfunctioning, or abnormal or disorganized peristalsis. The most common cause of gastroparesis is abnormal neurologic function of the nerves innervating the stomach; diabetes mellitus is typically the most frequent disorder noted.

Gastroparesis

Other causes of delayed gastric emptying include postoperative gastric surgery, Parkinson disease, and medications such as narcotic pain medications. Symptoms of gastroparesis may include feeling full after only a few bites (most common during a meal or immediately after a meal), nausea and vomiting, ill-defined stomach discomfort, and weight loss secondary to diminished appetite. Patients with diabetes may have wide swings in blood sugar secondary to the unpredictability of gastric emptying; gastroparesis should be suspected in patients with diabetes who have increasingly labile blood sugars. Diagnostic testing for gastroparesis can include endoscopy, upper GI series with barium swallow, and radioisotope gastric emptying scan.

Dietary treatment of gastroparesis may involve ingesting frequent small meals that contain minimal amounts of fat, fiber, and roughage. Liquid diets are typically easier for patients with gastroparesis. In patients with diabetes, tight blood sugar control may aid in improving and decreasing the symptoms of gastroparesis. Pro-motility medications such as metoclopramide facilitate gastric emptying in patients with gastroparesis. Erythromycin may also be utilized as a medication to treat delayed gastric emptying. Domperidone is a pro-motility medication that is widely used outside the United States but requires special approval from the FDA to be used in the United States.

Anti-emetic medications such as prochlorperazine and trimethobenzamide treat delayed gastric emptying by decreasing the symptoms of nausea and/or vomiting. Extreme weight loss associated with delayed gastric emptying may require the insertion of a feeding tube into the small intestine. New treatments under evaluation to treat the symptoms of gastroparesis include injection of botulinum toxin into the pylorus musculature in order to facilitate muscle relaxation and to improve emptying of the stomach. Implanting a pacemaker in the stomach to provide electrical stimulation of the stomach musculature has been used as well.

Cyclic Vomiting Syndrome

Cyclic vomiting syndrome is also known as CVS and is characterized by recurrent episodes of nausea and vomiting that are associated with symptom-free time periods. Patients with CVS seem to have a similar pattern for the episodes of vomiting. Symptoms of CVS are characterized by four episodic phases. The first phase is called the inter-episodic phase and is characterized by symptom-free periods of time that may last from weeks to months. The next phase is called the pre-emesis phase; the emetic phase is next; and the recovery phase is the last phase.

Many patients with CVS are often misdiagnosed or have delayed diagnosis. CVS is most commonly misdiagnosed as viral gastroenteritis. The Rome III study group on functional gastrointestinal disorders recently established criteria for the diagnosis of CVS. "The following 3 criteria must be fulfilled for the last 3 months with symptom onset at least 6 months before diagnosis:

- Stereotypical episodes of vomiting regarding onset (acute and duration less than 1 week);
- Three or more discrete episodes in the prior year; and
- Absence of nausea and vomiting between episodes.

Supportive criteria for the diagnosis of CVS include a history or family history of migraine headaches."

The typical treatment for CVS is largely based upon clinical expertise and experience with the disorder. Lifestyle alterations, such as eliminating factors that seem to trigger episodes, are important in CVS patients. Medication treatment is useful to allow for the prevention of subsequent episodes of CVS. It is also vital to use abortive measures and supportive measures in the midst of an acute flare-up of CVS. Good family and social support is also an essential element in the management of the disorder. It has been suggested that patients with CVS request a letter from their physician to present in the event of an emergency department visit.

Dumping Syndrome

Dumping syndrome is the term that is used to describe the symptoms of rapid gastric emptying that result in the small intestine receiving large boluses of undigested food, which inhibits proper absorption of nutrition. The most common cause of dumping syndrome is previous gastrectomy. The symptoms of dumping syndrome may include nausea, abdominal cramping, dizziness, diarrhea, weakness, and diaphoresis that happens during or after ingestion of food. The symptoms are characterized by early symptoms and by late symptoms. The early symptoms often happen during eating or after eating while the late symptoms occur 1-3 hours post-ingestion.

Commonly, the diagnosis of dumping syndrome is made based upon symptom occurrence in patients with a history of prior gastric surgery. It is important to consider using diagnostic testing to rule out other disorders. Diagnostic testing may include laboratory tests, upper GI endoscopy, and gastric emptying testing. Gastric emptying testing will show fast gastric emptying in the early scans visualized at a half-hour and an hour after ingestion of the test meal. Typically, the early post-ingestion scans will exhibit almost complete stomach emptying. Treatment may include dietary modifications and medications.

Dietary modifications for dumping syndrome are numerous and include ingesting smaller and more frequent meals; careful chewing and swallowing with an upright posture after eating; decreased solid food intake; liquid ingestion prior to or after meals; avoiding nutritional supplement drinks and milkshakes; limiting sugar ingestion; eating complex carbohydrates and foods with a large amount of soluble fiber; increasing dietary fat and protein ingestion; and the limitation or the elimination of products that contain lactose. If patients do not improve with dietary changes, medications that delay gastric emptying may be used, such as acarbose and octreotide.

Functional Dyspepsia

Functional dyspepsia is considered to be a gastric motility disorder and is often misdiagnosed as heartburn, IBS, GERD, functional gastrointestinal bloating, and functional biliary disorder. Functional dyspepsia is typically a clinical diagnosis. Symptoms of functional dyspepsia are differentiated into three categories: ulcer-like, dysmotility-like, and unspecified. Ulcer-like functional dyspepsia is most commonly associated with upper abdominal pain that is nocturnal, episodic, sometimes alleviated with food or antacids, and located in the upper mid abdomen. Dysmotility-like functional dyspepsia is usually accompanied by abdominal discomfort that is associated with early fullness, nausea/vomiting, and bloating.

Enteral Nutrition

Patients with acute and chronic illness often require nutritional support. Indicators of the need for nutritional support are malnutrition (most common), poor oral intake (which causes glycogen store depletion, gluconeogenesis, peripheral lipolysis, and amino acid breakdown in muscle), and severe multi-organ system disease (e.g., renal, liver, cardiac, respiratory, GI, or hematologic). Enteral and parenteral nutritional support may be utilized; however, enteral nutrition has many advantages over parenteral nutrition, such as being more cost-effective, improved maintenance of the integrity of the gut, decreased rates of infection, and a reduced length of the hospital stay.

Contraindications

There is an adage, "if the gut works, use it." Enteral nutritional support is typically the more favored method but has contraindications which include a lack or absence of intestinal function (may be secondary to intestinal failure, profound inflammation, or postoperative ileus/stasis), total intestinal obstruction, failure or impaired ability to utilize the gut for access for enteral nutritional support (an example would be in a severely burned patient), the presence of intestinal fistulae that cause high loss, and the ethical aspects of nutritional support in the dying or terminally ill patient.

Types of Access

It is important to assess the following patient aspects when choosing a device for access for enteral nutrition: the anatomy and the functional ability of the patient's GI tract, the projected length of time necessary for the use of enteral nutrition, and potential for the risk of aspiration. The most common device that is utilized for the administration of enteral nutrition is the nasogastric tube, which may be placed into the stomach, duodenum, or the jejunum. A lessened risk of aspiration is seen with NG tubes that are situated past the ligament of Treitz.

NG tubes are typically used in a patient that will need enteral nutrition for only a short period of time (usually less than 4 weeks); however, if the patient will need enteral nutritional support for a long period of time (typically more than 4 weeks), it is advisable to utilize a more permanent enteral nutrition device such as gastrostomy or jejunostomy tube. The gastrostomy tube is most commonly utilized for long-term enteral nutritional support. Gastrostomy insertion may be performed in a percutaneous manner (percutaneous endoscopic gastrostomy or PEG), under fluoroscopy, or surgically.

PEG Placement Techniques

The PEG tube is typically a more cost-effective option than surgical placement. The following PEG placement techniques are often used: Gauderer-Ponsky (pull), Sachs-Vine (push), Russell (introducer), Versa (T-fastener), and the primary button method. Possible complications of PEG tube placement can include major complications (1-4% of patients) and minor complications (4-33% of patients). Major complications of PEG tube placement include necrotizing fasciitis, buried bumper syndrome, colocutaneous fistula formation, accidental removal of the PEG tube, and aspiration into the pulmonary tree. Minor complications include peristomal infection/leakage, pneumoperitoneum, ileus, bleeding, ulceration, and tube clogging/dysfunction.

Placement of the Jejunal Feeding Tube

Jejunal feeding tubes may either be placed endoscopically or in a surgical manner. A jejunal feeding tube or J tube may be fed via endoscopy through an existing PEG tube (known as PEG/J). Endoscopy may also be used to place the J tube in a technique called percutaneous endoscopic jejunostomy or PEJ. This technique requires a direct small bowel puncture under percutaneous endoscopy. PEJ placement necessitates extra training; the small bowel is difficult to puncture since it often migrates away from the abdominal wall. Complications include infection, small intestinal abscess, and wound infection.

Surgical Placement of Feeding Tubes

Surgical placement of feeding tubes is typically indicated for patients that cannot safely have PEG or endoscopic feeding tube placement. Examples of such patients include those with obstruction from a tumor or those who are scheduled for other surgical procedures anyway. Surgical placement of feeding tubes may be either temporary or permanent. Temporary surgical feeding tube placement may be performed in a laparoscopic manner. The most common and preferred surgical technique that is utilized for tube feeding after major GI surgery is the needle catheter jejunostomy. Complications include tube obstruction, wound infection, tube leak, or accidental removal of the tube.

Polymeric Commercial Enteral Formulas

Commercial enteral formulas are characterized by the following four groups: polymeric, oligomeric, elemental, and special formulas. Polymeric formulas are considered to be nutritionally complete and have the following: whole protein (nitrogen source), oligosaccharides, maltodextrins or starch (carbohydrate source), fat source (usually vegetable oil), minerals, vitamins, and trace elements. These formulas will necessitate some form of digestion and of absorption. Polymeric formulas do not have lactose and may also be taken as an oral supplementation. The typical calorie density is 1 kcal/ml and is isotonic, but also can be concentrated to 1.5-2 kcal/ml.

Oligomeric Formulas

Oligomeric formulas are typically utilized in patients with impaired digestion or absorption. Examples of such patients are those with Crohn disease, short bowel syndrome, exocrine pancreatic insufficiency, fistulae, and radiation enteritis. Oligomeric formulas are composed of dipeptides, tripeptides, and free amino acids that are a nitrogen source that does not need intraluminal hydrolysis but can use active transport mechanisms for absorption. The fat source for oligomeric formulas is long-chain or medium-chain triglycerides. Oligomeric formulas also are composed of carbohydrates, minerals, vitamins, and trace elements. Oligomeric formulas are also considered to be complete nutritionally and have a low osmolality.

Elemental Formulas

Elemental commercial enteral formulas are composed of amino acids, monosaccharides, disaccharides, and fat in the form of medium-chain triglycerides or essential fatty acids. The caloric density of elemental commercial enteral formulas is 1 kcal/ml. The concentration of nitrogen in an elemental commercial enteral formula is 6-8 g/liter. Elemental commercial enteral formulas comprise many small particles. The presence of numerous small particles in elemental enteral formulas causes elemental formulas to have a high osmotic load. The osmotic load is in the range of 500-900 mOsm/l, which may yield osmotic diarrhea.

Modular Diets

Special enteral formulas may include modular diets. Modular diets can be a diet in which a single macronutrient can be administered. With a modular diet the type and amount of nutrients may be modified according to the needs of the patient. The modular diet is composed of carbohydrate, fat, and protein modules. Modular diets are used in patients with renal failure, cardiac failure, acid-base dysfunction, and electrolyte dysfunction. Modules of carbohydrates are utilized for patients who require an increased caloric intake; protein modules are utilized to provide an increased nitrogen intake; and fat modules are used to elevate energy intake and to provide essential fatty acids.

Special Formulas

Chronic hepatic disease can result in elevated levels of aromatic chain amino acids and lowered levels of branched chain amino acids, which can yield hepatic encephalopathy by the formation of false neurotransmitters. In patients with chronic hepatic disease, diets that are enriched with branched-chain amino acids and that are limited in aromatic amino acids are widely utilized. However, recent randomized and controlled trials have demonstrated that hepatic diets that are composed of increased branched-chain amino acids and decreased aromatic amino acids are useful only in hepatic encephalopathy that is not responsive to medication.

Patients with acute renal failure require the reduction of toxin accumulation; decreased serum urea nitrogen; and the maintenance of fluid, electrolyte, and nutritional balance. If a patient with acute renal failure is malnourished or in a hypercatabolic state, 1.5-1.8 grams of protein per kilogram of weight per day will be needed. Patients with chronic renal failure exhibit impaired ability to eliminate urea and electrolytes (primary contributors to the solute load of the kidney). In patients with CRF who are not on dialysis typically need low protein with increased essential amino acids, while patients with who are on dialysis need 1.2-1.3 g/kg of body weight of protein per day.

Other special formulas include pulmonary formulas, immune-enhancing formulas, formulas for GI dysfunction, and diabetic formulas. Pulmonary formulas are usually composed of modified carbohydrates and fat, since metabolism of a carbohydrate calorie yields more carbon dioxide than the metabolism of a fat calorie. However, most pulmonary patients with CO_2 retention are not given such formulas and have their energy intake at or below their needed levels for management. Immune-enhancing formulas are typically composed of glutamine, arginine, omega-3 fatty acids, nucleotides, and branched-chain fatty acids to provide increased resistance to infection.

Complications

Complications of enteral nutrition can be characterized as gastrointestinal (30-38%), mechanical (2-10%), metabolic, and infectious. GI complications include "abdominal cramping, Abdominal distension, nausea and vomiting, gastroesophageal reflux, diarrhea, malabsorption, GI bleeding, and ileus." Mechanical complications of enteral nutrition include "rhinitis, otitis, parotitis, pharyngitis, esophagitis, pulmonary aspiration, erosions of the esophagus, tube dislodgement, tube obstruction, and perforation." Metabolic and infectious complications of enteral nutrition include calcium, magnesium, and phosphorus disturbances; alterations in fluid and electrolyte balances; hyperosmolar conditions; hyperglycemia or hypoglycemia; bacterial or other microbial contamination; and bacterial colonization or infection.

GI Endocrine Tumors

The majorities of the cancerous tumors of the GI tract is either adenocarcinomas or squamous cell carcinomas and are of an endodermal epithelial origin. Some tumors of the GI tract are comprised of cells from the endocrine that originate from the neural crest, neuroectoderm, and the endoderm. The neuroendocrine system has neuroendocrine cells from the adrenal medulla, pancreatic islets, paraganglia, parathyroid, pituitary, and thyroid C cells and other neuroendocrine cells that are found throughout the body (GI tract, biliary tract, liver, lung, urethra, and skin). The majority of neuroendocrine tumors occur in the gastropancreatic axis (GEP).

Epidemiology

Neuroendocrine tumors make up 1.2-1.5% of all GI neoplasms; the incidence of new cases is 1.6-2.0 cases per 100,000 persons annually. In one institution, most cases of neuroendocrine GI tumors involved the rectum (51.9%), the stomach (21.9%), the duodenum (11.2%), the colon (5.9%), the appendix (3.2%), the esophagus (3.2%), and various other locations in the small intestine (2.1%). The majority of neuroendocrine tumors in the GI tract are sporadic, which indicates a non-familial origin. However, some of these tumors arise as part of familial MEN1 or neurofibromatosis type 1.

Tumor Markers

A major advancement in the diagnosis of neuroendocrine tumors of the GI tract has been the use of immunohistochemical staining. Neuroendocrine cells have the following characteristics: "the presence of dense core granules ultra-structurally, and the expression of certain marker proteins (i.e., general neuroendocrine markers) such as chromogranin, synaptophysin, and neuron-specific enolase (NSE), as well as cell-type specific hormonal products such as peptide hormones and amines." Chromogranin A is demonstrated in most neuroendocrine neoplasms; therefore, this marker is thought to be the most significant marker in general use. Synaptophysin is also thought to be a good general marker.

Classifications

Neuroendocrine tumors are now classified into well-differentiated endocrine tumors, well-differentiated endocrine carcinomas, and poorly differentiated endocrine carcinomas. The classification of well-differentiated endocrine tumors shows benign or uncertain potential for malignant behavior. The classification of well-differentiated endocrine carcinoma exhibits low-grade malignant behavior. The classification of poorly differentiated endocrine carcinoma is characterized by high-grade malignant behavior. With regard to GI endocrine tumors, the term *carcinoid* is still utilized and refers to a well-differentiated endocrine tumor; the term *malignant carcinoid* is still used and refers to a well-differentiated endocrine tumor as well. Subdivisions in the classifications also are used.

Subdivisions in the Classification Scheme

The classification scheme for GI endocrine tumors also has subdivisions that are categorized upon the location and the biologic behavior of the tumors. Locations for tumors in the subdivisions include the stomach, duodenum, proximal jejunum, distal jejunum and ileum, appendix, colorectal, and pancreas. Other criteria include the size of the tumor, the extent of vascular invasion, mitotic activity, the degree of histologic differentiation, the presence of metastatic disease, and the involvement of organs that are in close proximity. The presence of hormonal activity that is common to other disease states is also noted.

Endocrine Tumors of the Stomach

Endocrine tumors of the stomach are quite rare and account for less than 1% of all gastric cancers. Well-differentiated gastric endocrine tumors are sub-classified into 3 groups: type 1 is associated with chronic atrophic gastritis/pernicious anemia (70-80%); type 2 is associated with Zollinger-Ellison syndrome with multiple endocrine neoplasia type 1 (MEN 1-5%); and type 3 is sporadic (15-20%). Type 1 and type 2 gastric endocrine tumors have hypergastrinemia, which leads to hyperplasia of the enterochromaffin cells and results in hyperplastic lesions and numerous small carcinoid tumors. Type 3 gastric endocrine tumors do not exhibit hypergastrinemia and are more aggressive.

Imaging

The majority of gastric endocrine tumors are directly visualized and diagnosed via endoscopy. The use of endoscopic ultrasound is undertaken for larger tumors, to assess the extent of gastric invasion. CT of the abdomen or MRI is utilized in type 1 and type 2 gastric endocrine tumors that are greater than 2 cm in diameter and for type 3 tumors to assess for metastatic disease. Most gastric endocrine tumors are vascular and thus are easily demonstrated with contrast. MRI is the preferred method in patients with contrast allergy or renal insufficiency.

Management

Type 1 and type 2 gastric endocrine tumors typically have an indolent course; if less than 2 cm in diameter, these tumors may be removed via endoscopy and need interval follow-up. The presence of tumors greater than 2 cm in diameter, recurrent tumors, or more than 6 polyps will require surgical removal. Antrectomy has been utilized in patients with tumor secondary to chronic atrophic gastritis. Somatostatin analogs have been utilized in patients with type 2 tumors secondary to Zollinger-Ellison syndrome/multiple endocrine neoplasia 1 (MEN 1). Type 3 tumor usually requires a partial gastrectomy with lymph node dissection.

It is sometimes suggested for the younger patient who lacks risk factors and who has an unresectable metastatic gastric endocrine tumor that liver transplantation be performed. 5-15% of patients with metastatic liver disease with lesions that are localized to one lobe of the liver have been treated with hepatic resection. Hepatic resection in these patients has been shown to yield long-term relief of symptoms and improvement in survival time. Liver transplantation is currently controversial and is not routinely recommended. Embolization of the hepatic artery is sometimes used as a palliative treatment.

Upper GI Bleeding

Upper GI bleeding is defined as "bleeding derived from a source proximal to the ligament of Treitz." The incidence of upper GI bleeding is "100 cases per 100,000 population per year." Upper GI bleeding is approximately 4 times more common than lower GI tact bleeding; the mortality of upper GI bleeding is 6-10%. Upper GI bleeding that is nonvariceal in nature is caused by either arterial bleeding, mucosal tears (peptic ulcer disease), or low-pressure bleeding of a venous nature (telangiectasia and angiectasias). The cause of death in upper GI bleeding is typically comorbid illness rather than the actual hemorrhaging.

Peptic Ulcer Disease

The most common cause of upper GI bleeding is peptic ulcer disease, which is the cause of 27-40% of all cases. Risk factors for peptic ulcer disease include alcohol dependence, chronic renal failure, and nonsteroidal anti-inflammatory drugs. Peptic ulcer disease is strongly linked to *H. pylori* infection, which results in direct inflammatory injury to the mucosa of the stomach and duodenum, decreased mucosal defenses, and backflow of gastric acid. Treating *H. pylori* infection has decreased the risk of recurrent ulcer and recurrent GI bleeding. Duodenal ulcers are more common than gastric ulcers. However, the bleeding risk is the same for both duodenal and gastric ulcers. Hemorrhage is typically secondary to erosion of the artery in the bottom of the ulcer; 80% of patients with upper GI bleeding have spontaneous cessation of bleeding. Primary attempts at endoscopic hemostasis have a large failure rate. Patients who are at greater risk of re-bleeding after endoscopic treatment include age over 60, being in shock, a history of coagulopathy, the presence of active pulsatile hemorrhage, and cardiovascular disease.

Other Causes

Other causes of upper GI bleeding include mucosal tears of the esophagus or the fundus of the stomach (Mallory-Weiss tear), erosive gastritis, erosive esophagitis, Dieulafoy lesion, gastric carcinoma, and a gastric leiomyoma that ulcerates. Rare causes of upper GI bleeding include aortoenteric fistula, vascular ectasia of the antrum of the stomach, angiectasias, and Osler-Weber-Rendu syndrome. An aortoenteric fistula is secondary to the erosion of an aortic graft into the bowel lumen and typically occurs at the proximal aortic anastomotic suture line. Upper GI bleeding may also be due to acute stress gastritis.

Epidemiology and Prognosis

In the United States, 100,000 patients require hospital admission each year for the treatment of upper GI bleeding. The incidence of upper GI bleeding is twice as great in men as in women but the mortality rate is the same in both. The mortality from upper GI bleeding is greater in both men and women over age over 60 years. The mortality rate in patients over age 60 ranges from 12-25%. In patients 21-31 years of age, the mortality rate is 3.3%; patients 41-50 years of age have a mortality rate of 10.1%; and patients 71-80 years of age have a mortality rate of 14.4%.

Vascular Disorders of the GI Tract

There are two main divisions of vascular disorders of the GI tract, neoplastic and non-neoplastic. Neoplastic vascular disorders of the GI tract include endothelial cell tumors (hemangiomas and angiosarcomas, for example) and vascular tumors (Kaposi sarcoma and hemangiopericytomas, for example). Non-neoplastic vascular disorders of the GI tract include inflammatory (vasculitis, for example), obstructive (ischemic colitis, superior mesenteric ischemia, and chronic mesenteric ischemia, for example), and structural (venous-varices, hemorrhoids, capillary-gastric antral vascular ectasia, portal gastropathy, arteriovenous-angiodysplasia, telangiectasia, and arterial-Dieulafoy lesion, Ehlers-Danlos syndrome, pseudoxanthoma elasticum). The most common cause of small intestinal bleeding in patients over age 60 is angiodysplasia.

Angiodysplasia

Angiodysplasia is the cause of 5-6% of GI bleeds and is typically located in the upper or lower GI tract. 1% of patients having colonoscopy will be found to have asymptomatic angiodysplasia. Angiodysplasia is found primarily in the stomach in the upper GI tract and in the right colon in the lower GI tract. The lesions of angiodysplasia are located in the mucosa and the sub-mucosa of the bowel wall and are composed of veins, capillaries, and arteries that are dilated, thin-walled, and have endothelium with only a little smooth muscle.

Endoscopic Diagnosis and Therapy

Endoscopy is an important tool in the diagnosis of angiodysplasia. It should be remembered that angiodysplasia may cause chronic iron-deficiency anemia that makes the lesions more difficult to detect. In addition, meperidine should not be used for sedation because it will make the lesions of angiodysplasia seem to disappear. The lesions of angiodysplasia will appear "cherry-red" and have small radiating vessels and may look to be surrounded by a "pale halo sign." One of the favored endoscopic methods of treatment of angiodysplasia is to use argon plasma coagulation that is administered from the periphery in to the lesion.

Dieulafoy Lesion

The Dieulafoy lesion is an arterial vascular disorder wherein sub-mucosal end arteries are unusually large. This lesion may contribute to massive hemorrhage that may be fatal and is typically found in the upper stomach, 5-7 cm below the gastro-esophageal junction. These lesions have also been found in the distal stomach, the duodenum, and in the large intestine. The lesion is considered to be of congenital origin and occurs in 1.5% of patients with upper GI bleeding (primarily elderly men). The symptoms of a Dieulafoy lesion include hematemesis, hematochezia, melena, hypotension, and tachycardia.

Gastric Antral Vascular Ectasia (GAVE)

Gastric antral vascular ectasia (GAVE) is also known as "watermelon stomach." GAVE is a capillary vascular lesion wherein the antrum exhibits dilated and twisted mucosal capillaries that are often filled with thrombosis as well as dilated and twisted veins in the sub-mucosa. The antral wall appears thickened. Upon endoscopy, there are longitudinal parallel streaks that end at the pylorus and give the appearance of a watermelon. The exact etiology of GAVE is not known, GAVE is 5 times more common in women than in men. Patients with GAVE exhibit iron-deficiency anemia. It has been associated with hepatic cirrhosis, bone marrow transplants, scleroderma, and hypochlorhydria.

Hereditary Hemorrhagic Telangiectasia (HHT-Osler-Weber-Rendu Disease)

There is a distinction between angiodysplasia and telangiectasia. Telangiectasia is a term that denotes vascular lesions that are similar to those of angiodysplasia, but is part of a syndrome or a systemic disease process. Hereditary hemorrhagic telangiectasia is also known as Osler-Weber-Rendu disease and is characterized by telangiectasia involving the GI tract, nose, mouth, tongue, and lips. It is a rare autosomal dominant disease that can result in significant bleeding.

Small Intestine

Malabsorption

Malabsorption involves disorders and defects that are exhibited upon the digestion and absorption of food and nutrients in the GI tract and by infections in the GI tract. Malabsorption may be of only one element or may be diffuse. An example of a single defect is lactose intolerance; an example of diffuse defects is celiac disease or Crohn disease. The symptoms of malabsorption typically include diarrhea and weight loss. Treatment is commonly based upon delineating a specific etiology for the malabsorption such as celiac disease, Crohn disease, infection, or lactase deficiency.

Normal Physiology of Digestion and Absorption

Normal physiologic digestion and absorption in the intestinal system has three major aspects: luminal, mucosal, and post-absorptive. In the luminal phase, the hydrolysis of dietary fats, proteins, and carbohydrates occurs with the subsequent dissolving by bile and digestive enzymes. The brush border membrane of the epithelial cells of the intestine is crucial to the mucosal phase for transport of the resultant products of digestion from the lumen into cells. Lipids and essential nutrients are reassembled and travel by way of the lymphatics and the hepatic circulation from the epithelial cells to the rest of the body.

Clinical Presentation

Patients with malabsorption have a history of the following symptoms that are due to the osmotic load that is a consequence of the defect in absorption: diarrhea, steatorrhea, weight loss and fatigue, flatulence and bloating, edema, anemia, bleeding diatheses, skeletal metabolic defects, and neurologic symptoms. Diarrhea is the most common reported symptom in malabsorption and is characterized as watery and can result in profound dehydration. Steatorrhea reflects issues with fat absorption and is characterized by large light-colored stools with a significant odor. The patient often will note that his stool floats and is hard to flush.

Methane and hydrogen are generated through bacterial fermentation of the food that is not absorbed, which causes flatulence and abdominal bloating. Edema is due to the loss of albumin from chronic malabsorption of protein or is due to protein loss into the lumen of the intestine. Anemia is either microcytic (secondary to iron deficiency) or macrocytic (secondary to vitamin B_{12} deficiency). The malabsorption of vitamin K results in bleeding disorders, while the lack of vitamin D causes metabolic defects in the skeleton. Electrolyte deficiencies may yield neurologic issues such as tetany, while vitamin lack may cause neuropathy.

Causes

The causes of malabsorption are usually classified upon the basis of the three phases of digestion and absorption. Luminal phase causes of malabsorption include impaired nutrient hydrolysis, micelle formation defects, and luminal availability and processing. Defective nutrient hydrolysis is most often due to pancreatic issues such as chronic pancreatitis, resection of the pancreas, cancer of the pancreas, and cystic fibrosis. A lack or decreased level of lipase and proteases results in the malabsorption of lipids and proteins. Gastric hypersecretion (Zollinger-Ellison syndrome) causes the inactivation of pancreatic enzymes as well.

Other causes of defective nutrient hydrolysis in the luminal phase of digestion and absorption may be a result of impaired mixing of nutrients, bile enzymes, and pancreatic enzymes from disorders like rapid intestinal transit (dumping syndrome); postoperative gastrojejunostomy; gastrectomy (both partial gastrectomy and total gastrectomy); mesenteric thrombosis or embolus; and subsequent intestinal removal. Defects in the conversion of pro-enzymes to active forms of enzymes may result in impaired nutrient hydrolysis. Deficiencies of enterokinase and trypsinogen will cause resultant impaired hydrolysis of nutrients in the form of protein malabsorption and maldigestion.

Defective micelle formation results in issues with the solubilization of fats, which causes fat malabsorption. Defects in the formation of micelles are the result of a lack of bile salt synthesis as seen in parenchymal hepatic disease (cirrhosis); defective secretion of bile as a result of cholestatic jaundice (primary biliary cirrhosis or primary sclerosing cholangitis) or biliary obstruction; defects in entero-hepatic bile circulation (post-operative small bowel resection or regional enteritis); or an overgrowth of bacteria in the small intestine, causing the deconjugation of bile salts. Other causes include disorders that result in stasis of material in the small intestine.

Review Video: Lactose Intolerance
Visit mometrix.com/academy and enter code: 672651

Mucosal Phase

Defective brush border hydrolase function causes malabsorption in the mucosal phase and may be a result of the following conditions: disaccharidase deficiency—lactase deficiency is the most common (primary lactase deficiency is genetic, while secondary lactase deficiency is due to rotavirus, Giardia, alcoholism, celiac sprue, radiation and regional enteritis, or AIDS enteropathy); immunoglobulin A deficiency (most common and presents with symptoms like celiac disease); acrodermatitis enteropathica (autosomal recessive, causing defective zinc absorption); and autoimmune enteropathy (intractable secretory diarrhea and atrophy of the villi due to antibodies that are formed against intestinal epithelial and goblet cells).

Post-Absorptive Phase

The causes of defective nutrient absorption may be primary or acquired. Primary disorders of nutrient absorption are inherited and include glucose-galactose malabsorption, abetalipoproteinemia, cystinuria, and Hartnup disease. Acquired disorders of nutrient absorption include intestinal resection or bypass (resulting in less of an absorptive surface area); injury or damage to the absorbing surface of the intestine (celiac sprue, tropical sprue, Crohn disease, AIDS enteropathy, chemotherapy or radiation therapy); infiltrative (lymphoma, amyloidosis); and infections. Post-absorptive phase causes include lymphatic system obstruction, which may be primary or acquired. Primary causes include intestinal lymphangiectasia and Milroy disease.

Diagnostic Work-Up

Laboratory tests are important in the diagnostic work-up of malabsorption. Hematologic studies include CBC: microcytic anemia due to iron deficiency or macrocytic anemia due to vitamin B_{12} or folate deficiency; serum iron, vitamin B_{12}, and folate levels; and elevated prothrombin time due to vitamin K deficiency. Chemistries include electrolytes to detect low levels of potassium, calcium, magnesium, and metabolic acidosis; protein and albumin levels; lipid panel to detect decreased levels of triglycerides, cholesterol, alpha- and beta-carotene; and a sedimentation rate to detect Crohn disease and Whipple disease. Serology includes testing for IgA deficiency.

A small bowel series with barium swallow may demonstrate the following abnormalities: an abnormal small intestinal pattern may yield the cause of malabsorption; celiac disease may exhibit a coarse or even obliterated mucosal pattern; barium flocculation may be noted in the lumen of the gut; scleroderma may exhibit dilation of the small intestine with diverticulosis; the presence of stricture, fistula, or ulceration may be the result of regional enteritis; and postoperative changes or enterocolonic fistula may also be noted. CT of the abdomen may identify chronic pancreatitis, Whipple disease, or lymphoma. ERCP may identify pancreatic or biliary issues causing malabsorption.

Tests for fat malabsorption include 72-hour fecal fat collection, acid steatocrit, and Sudan III stain of the stool. If a 72-hour fecal fat collection exhibits malabsorption, a D-xylose test may then be done to assess the integrity of the mucosa of the intestine. If the D-xylose test reveals low urinary levels of D-xylose, a factor involving the intestinal lumen or the absorptive surface area may be present. Carbohydrate malabsorption may be tested with a hydrogen breath test; a bile salt breath test may be used to determine bile salt absorption. A Schilling test aids in determining the nature of vitamin B_{12} deficiency. Upper GI endoscopy with biopsy may also be used.

MANAGEMENT AND TREATMENT

It is vital to identify treatable causes of malabsorption, if possible, and to eliminate nutritional deficiencies. Management of nutrition includes supplementation of minerals such as calcium, magnesium, iron, and various vitamins; and replenishment of protein and calories. Medium-chain triglycerides should be used as substitutes for fats, since medium-chain triglycerides do not need the formation of micelles for their absorption and utilize a portal transport mechanism as opposed to a lymphatic transport mechanism. Parenteral nutrition may be necessary in situations like extensive intestinal resection and diffuse or massive regional enteritis. Specific diets and enzyme supplements may also be needed.

SMALL INTESTINE BACTERIAL OVERGROWTH (BOS)

Bacterial overgrowth syndrome or BOS is the term for a clinical syndrome in which the normal level of bacteria in the small intestine increases to a large amount, or in which the normal flora is replaced by pathogenic bacteria. The upper GI tract and the small intestine normally have a low level of symbiotic bacteria that are necessary for normal digestive processes, development of the intestine, and immunity. Typical species of such bacteria include *lactobacilli*, *enterococci*, oral *streptococci*, and other forms of gram-positive aerobes or facultative anaerobes. There are numerous etiologies for the overgrowth of bacteria.

NORMAL PHYSIOLOGY

The normal bacterial and fungal colony count in the duodenum and the jejunum is less than 100,000 organisms/ml; anaerobic bacteria are not noted in the jejunum in normal patients. About 33% of aspirates of the jejunum are considered sterile. The ileum typically has less than 100,000,000 organisms/ml of aerobic and anaerobic bacteria. Bacterial colonization in various aspects of the GI tract differs due to peristalsis; pH; redox potential; the adhesion, cooperation, and antagonism of bacteria; the secretion of mucin; diet; and the availability of various nutrients. Peristalsis serves the protective function of clearing pathogenic bacteria from the small intestine.

OTHER PROTECTIVE FACTORS

Gastric acid and bile get rid of many potentially pathogenic bacteria prior to exiting the stomach. Enzymes in the intestine, pancreas, and biliary secretions aid in the destruction of unwanted bacteria in the small intestine. The intact mucosa of the gut and the layer of mucin also aid in protecting the gut from unwanted bacteria. The production and secretion of immunoglobulin and macrophages and lymphocytes are also gut-protective mechanisms. The normal bacteria of the intestine, such as *Lactobacillus*, aid in the prevention of overgrowth by establishing a low pH.

PATHOPHYSIOLOGY OF BACTERIAL OVERGROWTH

If the normal mechanisms of protection in the intestine are disrupted, bacterial overgrowth can be the result. Desynchronization of peristalsis may cause issues with overgrowth of bacteria. Anatomic defects like blind pouch formation may result in stagnation and overgrowth. If bile acids, fats, carbohydrates, proteins, and nutrients are not absorbed properly, the result may be direct injury to the lining of the lumen by bacteria or by the change of nutrients into toxic compounds; this may lead to the profound diarrhea and weight loss typically associated with bacterial overgrowth syndrome.

EPIDEMIOLOGY

The symptoms of bacterial overgrowth syndrome are often also present in patients with other causes of malabsorption and conditions that cause diarrhea. Therefore, prevalence estimates are probably too low. For example, 20-43% of chronic diarrhea in patients with diabetics is due to BOS. Some neonatal patients (50% with chronic diarrhea have BOS) have a disruption of the normal protective mechanisms to alleviate bacterial overgrowth. The elderly population has a higher prevalence of BOS due to the decreased production of gastric acid and hypomotility from medications.

MORTALITY AND MORBIDITY

Bacterial overgrowth syndrome may contribute to increased problems that accompany malabsorption and chronic diarrhea. In certain patients, bacterial overgrowth syndrome may lead to increased morbidity or mortality. The following are examples of patient populations that exhibit greater mortality with bacterial overgrowth syndrome: neonates or infants with concomitant malabsorption, malnutrition, or inherited/congenital GI anomalies; elderly patients with numerous medical conditions and chronic diarrhea; patients who have had previous upper intestinal operations that disrupt the mechanisms for protection of the intestine from bacterial overgrowth; patients with concomitant malnutrition; and patients with diabetes or scleroderma whose underlying disorders are not properly treated.

SYMPTOMS

Most of the symptoms of bacterial overgrowth syndrome are nonspecific and are often seen in other GI disorders. Some of the more typical symptoms of bacterial overgrowth syndrome include bloating, flatulence, abdominal pain, diarrhea, dyspepsia, and weight loss. Findings of symptoms of malabsorption can suggest advanced cases of bacterial overgrowth syndrome and include microcytic anemia secondary to iron deficiency, macrocytic anemia secondary to vitamin B_{12} or folate deficiency, polyneuropathy secondary to vitamin B_{12} deficiency, steatorrhea as a result of lipid malabsorption, tetany (hypocalcemia), night blindness, dermatitis (low selenium), rosacea, and cachexia.

CAUSES

Various medical conditions or abnormalities in structure may impair the normal protective mechanisms that inhibit bacterial overgrowth. Medical conditions that may cause bacterial overgrowth syndrome include prior upper intestinal tract operation, irritable bowel syndrome, cirrhosis, celiac disease, immune system deficiency (e.g., AIDS, IgA deficiency, malnutrition), short-bowel syndrome, end-stage renal disease, gastrojejunal anastomosis, vagotomy (not associated with selective parietal cell vagotomy, however), antral resection, and a lack of pancreatic exocrine function. Altered small bowel motility from diabetic autonomic neuropathy, scleroderma, amyloidosis, pseudo-obstruction, myotonic dystrophy, Parkinson disease, radiation enteritis, Crohn disease, and hypothyroidism can also cause BOS. Certain conditions cause formation of blind pouches, which can lead to bacterial overgrowth syndrome and include anastomoses (side-to-side and end-to-side), intra-abdominal reservoirs, diverticula in the duodenum or the jejunum, segmental ileal dilatation, blind-loop syndrome, biliopancreatic diversion, and megacolon as a result of Chagas disease. The presence of a fistula, such as a gastrocolic fistula or a jejunal-colic fistula, causes improper intestinal communication leading to bacterial overgrowth. Certain conditions may cause a partial obstruction that leads to bacterial overgrowth and include adhesions, strictures, masses, and leiomyosarcoma. Decreased gastric acid from achlorhydria, vagotomy, or chronic PPI use also can cause BOS.

Differential Diagnosis

The differential diagnoses to consider for bacterial overgrowth syndrome are numerous and include the following: amebiasis, intestinal carcinoid tumor, celiac sprue, Crohn disease, cryptosporidiosis, Cyclospora, CMV, diverticulosis of the small intestine, Giardia infection, inflammatory bowel disease, intestinal fistula formation, disorders of intestinal motility, pseudo-obstruction of the intestine, irritable bowel syndrome, isosporiasis, lactose intolerance, malabsorptive syndromes, microsporidiosis, chronic pancreatitis, pneumatosis cystoides intestinalis, tropical sprue, ulcerative colitis, VIPomas, and Whipple disease. Appropriate diagnostic testing and work-up should be undertaken to rule out such disorders in the differential; diagnostic work-up may include specific laboratory tests, imaging studies, or procedures.

Diagnostic Work-Up

Laboratory testing for bacterial overgrowth syndrome should encompass a work-up for diarrhea, malabsorption, and anemia. Routine laboratory work-up of anemia and an evaluation of nutrition should also be performed. Stool testing may demonstrate a pH that is acidic as well as the presence of reducing substances. The levels of D-lactic acid can be obtained from either the urine or the serum; if elevated, they may be useful in ascertaining whether BOS is present or another metabolic condition is present. Short-chain fatty acid levels, keto-bile acid concentrations, and urine-4-hydroxyphenylacetic acid levels may also be measured.

Imaging studies such as a small bowel follow-through are useful to identify possible causes of structural or mobility impairment that lead to bacterial overgrowth such as mal-rotation, strictures, diverticulosis, fistulae, or pseudo-obstruction. The function of breath testing in the diagnosis of bacterial overgrowth syndrome is to quantitate the levels of the byproducts of bacterial metabolism in order to differentiate substances that are not absorbed properly. The hydrogen breath test is utilized because in healthy patients, hydrogen is produced solely from intestinal bacteria (anaerobic bacteria in the small intestine cause elevated levels in BOS).

The hydrogen breath test will show an early elevation of the concentration of hydrogen exhaled as fermenting bacteria that have caused overgrowth in the small intestine subsequently cause fermentation of carbohydrates. The hydrogen breath test typically requires giving 1-2 mg/kg of glucose (do not use more than 25-50 g); an elevation in exhaled hydrogen to 20 parts per million is diagnostic. The bile acid breath test uses glycocholate that is labeled with carbon 14; abnormal increases in radioactive carbon dioxide levels exhibit bacterial glycocholate deconjugation. The xylose breath test has been shown to give the best specificity.

Medical Treatment

Medical treatment in bacterial overgrowth syndrome must focus upon the underlying cause (if known), antibiotics, and nutritional supplementation. It is vital to first correct a primary disease process or structural defect that may be causing bacterial overgrowth. Often, a large number of the clinical disorders that cause bacterial overgrowth are not easily remedied; thus, antibiotic treatment is used in order to re-establish a more normal intestinal bacterial flora. It is crucial to recall that the antibiotic treatment should not eradicate protective/normal organisms. The initial antibiotic regimen should be broad-spectrum and cover both aerobes and anaerobes.

Antibiotics that are utilized in the treatment of BOS include amoxicillin-clavulanate (75% effective in patients with diabetes), rifaximin (eliminates bacterial overgrowth in 80% of cases, especially if due to irritable bowel syndrome as well); clindamycin and metronidazole are often used in the elderly population with idiopathic bacterial overgrowth. In the neonatal and infant population with intractable diarrhea, studies show that treatment with cholestyramine and gentamicin can greatly decrease stool weight after 4-5 days of treatment. In the majority of patients with bacterial overgrowth syndrome due to Crohn disease, ciprofloxacin and metronidazole have been effective.

GI Problems and HIV

GI problems and hepatobiliary disorders are some of the most typical symptoms in patients with HIV infection. The use of antiretroviral therapies has affected the course of HIV infection and has altered many of the GI manifestations of HIV infection. Before the use of antiretroviral therapies, approximately 90-93% of patients with HIV infection exhibited significant GI issues. Currently, studies demonstrate that utilizing antiretroviral therapies and prophylactic regimens for *Pneumocystis carinii*, *Mycobacterium avium*, and cytomegalovirus can delay the onset or prevent opportunistic infections of the GI tract. It is vital to uncover treatable causes and to relieve GI symptoms.

Symptoms

GI symptoms in patients with HIV infection are numerous and may include diarrhea, dysphagia, odynophagia, nausea, vomiting, weight loss, abdominal pain, anorectal diseases, jaundice, liver enlargement, GI bleeding, synergistic interaction with HIV and hepatotrophic viruses, and tumors of the GI tract (Kaposi sarcoma, non-Hodgkin lymphoma). When evaluating GI symptoms in patients with HIV infection, it is critical to focus upon the degree of immunosuppression present. A progression of the degree of immunocompromise in HIV infections typically manifests as increased GI symptoms and is typically an endpoint.

It is important to consider that opportunistic infections of the GI tract are not common in patients with a CD4 count above 200. The clinical signs and symptoms of GI disorders rarely point to a specific cause; therefore, it is important to utilize objective testing and diagnostic studies to pinpoint an infection that is treatable or to identify a neoplasm that is commonly seen in HIV infection. However, empiric treatment for esophageal candidiasis is usually undertaken prior to work-up. It is also crucial to recall that multiple GI infections may also be present.

Small-Bowel Overgrowth and AIDS Enteropathy

Small-bowel overgrowth or SBO is a clinical syndrome that presents with diarrhea and the malabsorption of fat, vitamin B_{12}, and carbohydrates. Histologic findings of villous atrophy and inflammatory infiltrates are like those seen in AIDS enteropathy. Clinical factors that contribute to SBO include lack of gastric acid, poor intestinal immunologic function, and impaired motility of the intestine. Research has shown that HIV may be an indirect pathogenic factor in causing diarrhea, since HIV viral proteins have been demonstrated in the intestinal tract. HIV may also contribute to impaired immunity and to impaired motility.

Diarrhea

Diarrhea is the most common symptom in patients with HIV infection. Diarrhea may be due to infections or neoplasms, or may be idiopathic in nature. Infectious causes can be bacterial, viral, or fungal. Bacterial causes include Mycobacterium avium-intracellulare, *Salmonella*, *Shigella*,

Campylobacter sp., *Clostridioides difficile*, small-bowel overgrowth, and *Vibrio parahaemolyticus*. Viral causes include CMV, herpes simplex, adenovirus, picobirnavirus, and HIV. Fungal causes include *Candida* and *Histoplasma capsulatum*. Neoplasms include Kaposi sarcoma and lymphoma. An idiopathic cause of diarrhea is AIDS enteropathy. MAC-diarrhea is uniquely associated with HIV infection. Early diarrhea in HIV infection is typically secondary to medications.

When evaluating diarrhea in HIV infection, it is crucial to obtain a thorough history that includes information regarding diet (lactose or fatty food intolerance), medications, cathartics (mega-doses of vitamin C, medications that contain lactose, or sorbitol ingestion, for example), and symptoms consistent with systemic infection or with neoplasms. Cramping, bloating, or nausea may indicate stomach or small bowel locale, which may be secondary to infections from *Cryptosporidium* or *Giardia*, for example. Hematochezia with tenesmus suggests large bowel involvement due to CMV, *Shigella*, *Campylobacter*, or *C. difficile* infections, for example.

The most imperative goal in evaluating diarrhea associated with HIV infection is to identify a treatable infection or neoplasm if possible. After diet and medications have been eliminated as possible causes of diarrhea, a stool culture for enteric bacteria should be obtained as well as *C. difficile* toxin and 3 stool samples to search for ova and parasites (include acid-fast bacilli and tri-chrome staining). Sigmoid examination is necessary if stool culture and stool samples do not reveal a diagnosis. Biopsies may be gotten from areas that appear abnormal or randomly if no obvious abnormalities are noted.

If the diarrhea in HIV infection is due to a specific pathogen, appropriate therapy should be started. A regimen of chronic and alternating antibiotics may be needed for treatment of recurrent *Salmonella*, *Shigella*, *Campylobacter*, and *Isospora* infections. Empiric treatment with antibiotics or with antiparasitics may be used for the chance of SBO syndrome, undiagnosed *Campylobacter* infection, *Isospora enteritis*, or undiagnosed protozoal infections. Examples of medications that are used in these situations can include sulfonamides, ciprofloxacin, tetracycline, and metronidazole. Chronic diarrhea in HIV infection may be treated with the use antidiarrheal medications.

Weight Loss

Weight loss is very common in advanced HIV infection with GI manifestations. The CDC defines wasting as an AIDS diagnosis "when a patient presents with involuntary weight loss of more than 10% of baseline body weight, plus either chronic diarrhea or chronic weakness and fever in the absence of infection or a condition other than HIV disease." With continued weight loss, death always results when the body weight goes below 66% of the ideal body weight. There are two etiologies of weight loss seen in HIV infection. Two etiologies have been demonstrated in involuntary weight loss associated with HIV infection: caloric deficit and metabolic disturbance. Upper GI tract abnormalities (anorexia, nausea, and vomiting), psychosocial issues, economic issues, fatigue, changes in mental status, and medications may result in caloric deficits that cause weight loss. Patients may choose to decrease intake to attempt to manage symptoms of diarrhea or of abdominal pain. In the setting of caloric deficit, the body will use fat stores as an energy source in order to protect lean body mass. Metabolic disturbances result in more energy expenditure or in an abnormal use of energy substrates.

Patients with weight loss and HIV infection need nutritional and functional evaluations. Advanced disease factors that may be able to be reversed include body composition alterations, exercise limitations, and functional limitations. Symptoms that result in poor intake and mechanisms to foster weight gain need to be addressed quickly. The following are indicators of issues with proper intake: anorexia, early satiety, nausea, vomiting, weakness, fatigue, odynophagia, dysphagia, dental issues, diarrhea, and abdominal pain. The following may indicate an increase in energy expenditure: fever, tachypnea, systemic infections, or increases in physical activity. Herbal supplements and lifestyle factors also need reviewed.

Nutritional management of weight loss in HIV infection strives to maintain lean body mass. Dietitians are essential team members in management who monitor weight status, body cell mass composition, caloric intake, and functional activity status levels. Three-day food logs are often used in order to assess true caloric intake. Protein needs, without the presence of infection, are 1-1.2 g/kg with a nutrient intake of 100% of the RDA. Supplementation with a multivitamin is also often necessary. Other means of management include appetite stimulants, nutritional supplements, and enteral/parenteral nutrition.

Abdominal Pain

Abdominal pain is frequently seen in patients with HIV infection and may indicate severe issues. It is important to consider infections, neoplasms, and even common etiologies of abdominal pain in HIV infection. The differential diagnosis for abdominal pain in HIV infection is usually grouped according to the location of the pain. Stomach location: gastritis or tumor (CMV or *Cryptosporidium*), ulcer (CMV or *Candida*), and outlet obstruction (*Cryptosporidium*, CMV, lymphoma). Small bowel location: enteritis (*Cryptosporidium*, MAC, or CMV), obstruction (Kaposi sarcoma or lymphoma), perforation (CMV or lymphoma). Colon location: colitis, obstruction, perforation, appendicitis.

Colitis is often caused by CMV, HSV, *Shigella*, and *Salmonella*, *Campylobacter*, or *C. difficile*. Obstruction in the colon is caused by lymphoma or *Kaposi* sarcoma. Perforation of the colon is due to CMV, lymphoma, or herpes simplex virus. Appendicitis may be the result of Kaposi sarcoma, CMV, MAC, *Cryptosporidium*. Pain in the location of the liver and/or spleen may be infiltrative (CMV, MAC, or lymphoma) or due to cholecystitis (CMV, *Cryptosporidium*, *Enterobacter*, or *Candida*), papillary stenosis (CMV, *Cryptosporidium*, Kaposi sarcoma), and cholangitis (CMV). Pain in the area of the pancreas is due to inflammation due to CMV, tuberculosis, MAC, and medications. Mesenteric infiltration is due to MAC, lymphoma, or KS. Pain in the peritoneum is due to vibrio and other causes.

Evaluation of abdominal pain in HIV infection should be the same work-up as for pain in the non-infected patient with the exception that US and CT scans should be obtained early to facilitate atypical regions as a location of the source of pain. Atypical findings may include abdominal wall thickening, gallbladder wall thickening, liver lesions, pancreatic lesions or infiltrations, etc. CMV infection usually results in perforation that occurs in the distal aspect of the small bowel or the colon. Obstruction may be the result of a neoplasm but may also be secondary to inflammation or stricture.

Peritonitis may be secondary to infection with histoplasmosis, tuberculosis, vibrio, MAC, and toxoplasmosis. Ascites may indicate the need for laparoscopic evaluation. Pancreatitis may be the cause of abdominal pain and will demonstrate high levels of amylase and of lipase. The most likely cause of pancreatitis in HIV infection is secondary to medications. The most common medications that contribute to pancreatitis in HIV infection are co-trimoxazole, pentamidine, and dideoxyinosine. Pancreatitis due to pentamidine can result from either IV administration or from inhaled administration. Pancreatitis may also be the result of infection from multiple organisms.

Pain Syndromes

The pain syndrome consisting of symptoms of dull pain, nausea, vomiting, and diarrhea is most likely due to infectious enteritis with diagnostic testing to confirm consistency of stool cultures, stool staining for ova and parasites, and sigmoid examination. The symptoms of severe acute pain and peritonitis are most commonly caused by perforation and should be confirmed by abdominal series with flat-plate and upright and have a surgical consult. The symptoms of RUQ pain and abnormal LFTs are most likely secondary to cholecystitis, cholangitis, or hepatic infiltration and should be confirmed by US/CT, ERCP, or liver biopsy. Subacute pain with profound nausea/vomiting may indicate obstruction and should be confirmed by radiographs and contrast.

GI Bleeding

GI bleeding in HIV infection typically occurs in less than 1% of patients and is often secondary to causes that are commonly seen in patients without HIV, such as peptic ulcer, stress ulcer, variceal hemorrhage, inflammatory bowel disease, polyps, diverticular disease, and cancer. Some infectious diseases and neoplasms unique to HIV infection may cause GI bleeding. CMV infection of the GI tract may result in ischemia or infarction in the distal small bowel or colon and lead to hemorrhage. Erosive esophagitis with hemorrhage is rarely seen with *Candida* infection of the esophagus.

A very rare cause of esophageal hemorrhage is late-stage HSV infection, which may contribute to ulcerations of the mucosa that combine to yield diffuse hemorrhagic esophagitis. Most patients with HIV infection and Cryptosporidiosis primarily have diarrhea but some may have hematochezia associated with enteritis. Enteritis secondary to infection with *Shigella*, *Salmonella*, or *Campylobacter* may be associated with bloody watery diarrhea. Infections with *E. histolytica*, chlamydia, or histoplasmosis may result in colonic ulcerations that cause GI bleeding. HIV-associated neoplasms may rarely cause GI bleeding. Kaposi sarcoma is typically asymptomatic but may have spontaneous ulcerations that bleed.

Kaposi Sarcoma

GI manifestations of Kaposi sarcoma usually occur in late-stage HIV infection and may be demonstrated in 56-70% of patients with Kaposi sarcoma. Studies have shown that patients with a large number of skin lesions due to Kaposi sarcoma seem to be more likely to have GI Kaposi sarcoma. GI Kaposi sarcoma typically has widely disseminated lesions that are usually not symptomatic but can result in large bulky masses. Kaposi sarcoma may also involve the hepatobiliary system and is usually not symptomatic, unless biliary obstruction occurs secondary to involvement of the distal common bile duct.

Lymphoma

There has been a tremendous increase in the incidence of non-Hodgkin lymphoma in patients with advanced HIV infection. The tumors are typically of B cell origin and are of high grade. Involvement of the GI tract or the hepatobiliary system occurs with lymphoma in 27-74% of HIV patients with lymphoma. Most HIV patients with lymphoma will present with extra-nodal disease; 33% have primary GI lymphoma or primary hepatobiliary tree lymphoma. The most commonly involved area is the hepatic parenchyma or the rectum. Such lymphomas are typically very aggressive in nature.

Review Video: Lymphoma
Visit mometrix.com/academy and enter code: 513277

Endocrine Tumors of the Small Intestine

Endocrine tumors of the small intestine originate in serotonin-producing intra-epithelial cells known as enterochromaffin cells. Most of the endocrine tumors of the small intestine are considered to be well differentiated but may exhibit various forms of biologic behavior. These small intestinal endocrine tumors possess amine precursor uptake and decarboxylation activity (APUD) which causes certain symptoms. Endocrine tumors are the most common of the small bowel cancers (41.8% of all small bowel neoplasms). These endocrine tumors are typically located in the ileum within 60 cm of the ileocecal valve. The average age for such tumors is between 55 and 60 years.

Clinical Presentation

Most patients with endocrine tumors of the small bowel typically do not have symptoms related to the tumor until hepatic metastases (which interfere with the liver's ability to metabolize humoral factors from the tumor) or obstruction/ischemia of the small bowel occurs. Therefore, most of the patients with an endocrine tumor of the small intestine have either regional or distant metastatic disease upon presentation. The most typical symptom is that of vague and colicky abdominal pain, which may be an indicator of small bowel obstruction secondary to mesenteric fibrosis or invasion.

Carcinoid Syndrome

5-7% of patients with an endocrine tumor of the small intestine have carcinoid syndrome. Carcinoid syndrome is secondary to the release of humoral factors from the tumor and is typically characterized by flushing (occurs in 75% of patients with carcinoid syndrome). Flushing as seen in carcinoid syndrome is usually diffuse and erythematous, and involves the face, neck, and upper thoracic region. It typically persists for 2-10 minutes and may be caused by stress, foods, or alcohol ingestion. 75-80% of patients with carcinoid experience watery diarrhea and cramping abdominal pain.

Cardiac Lesions

40% of patients with carcinoid syndrome develop cardiac lesions. The right heart is most typically affected, with thickening of the endocardium and pulmonic valve, and a tricuspid valve that is plaque-like in nature. This results in pulmonary stenosis, tricuspid stenosis, and tricuspid insufficiency. Other symptoms that are seen in patients with carcinoid syndrome secondary to small bowel endocrine tumor may include bronchoconstriction, wheezing (which occurs in 20% of those with carcinoid syndrome and is the least frequently seen symptom), and extensive hepatic metastases. The presence of carcinoid syndrome is typically considered a marker of advanced disease.

Biochemical Markers

A high level of 24-hour urinary 5-HIAA is utilized to confirm the diagnosis of carcinoid syndrome. The normal level for 24-hour urinary 5-HIAA is from 2-8 mg/day; levels of 30 mg/day may be seen secondary to certain medications, foods that are high in tryptophan, celiac disease, and Whipple disease. Carcinoid patients will usually have levels of 24-hour urinary 5-HIAA of over 100 mg/day. Chromogranins are stored proteins that are released in conjunction with peptide and amine humoral factors and are made in increased levels by small intestinal endocrine tumors.

Use of Chromogranin A and Whole-Blood Serotonin Concentration as Markers

Chromogranin A is sensitive but not specific for endocrine tumors of the small bowel. Plasma chromogranin A levels over 32 U/l are 75% sensitive and 84% specific for carcinoid syndrome. A plasma chromogranin level greater than 5000 micrograms/l is an independent marker that indicates dismal overall survival rates in carcinoid syndrome. Levels of chromogranin A have been correlated with the extent of the tumor burden present and are useful to monitor for the recurrence of tumor. False-positive levels of chromogranin A can be seen with hepatic, renal, and cardiac failure.

Imaging Studies

CT scan is commonly utilized in the diagnosis of carcinoid tumors but may not successfully demonstrate a small primary small intestinal endocrine tumor. The CT scan is helpful in the delineation of large and bulky lymph node and hepatic metastases. Tumors with hepatic metastases are typically hypervascular and will appear hypodense when compared to normal hepatic parenchyma after contrast. Another imaging study that is useful in the diagnosis of small bowel endocrine tumors is somatostatin receptor scintigraphy (SRS), which is primarily utilized to determine the extent of metastatic disease. Over 90% of carcinoid tumors possess large amounts of somatostatin receptors.

Treatment

An exploratory laparotomy is typically required in order to identify the primary tumor and to run the small intestine in its entirety, because 30% of patients will have synchronous endocrine tumors. The mesentery of the small intestine is scrutinized for enlarged lymph nodes, and the liver is examined for metastatic disease. An intraoperative hepatic ultrasound is often useful in demonstrating the extent of hepatic metastasis. 33% of patients with endocrine tumors of the small bowel will also have hepatic metastases. The potential for metastases is determined by the size of the primary tumor.

Surgical Treatment

The surgical treatment of endocrine tumors of the small intestine requires removal of the primary tumor with a segmental resection of the small bowel that is involved, as well as the accompanying mesentery with careful attention to the margins of resection, the lymphatic drainage of the neoplasm, and the preservation of the vascular supply to the small bowel margins. The technique of utilizing isosulfan blue dye to map the subserosal channels is helpful intraoperatively, because this technique can aid in the determination of the adequacy of resection margins and in the preservation of the ileocecal valve.

Metastatic Disease

Even in patients with documented hepatic metastases, it is still recommended to remove the involved small intestine and the accompanying mesentery in order to decrease symptoms of abdominal pain, to prevent compromise of the blood supply, and to prevent small bowel obstruction. The majority of patients with endocrine tumors of the small bowel will need treatment with octreotide. Octreotide causes gallstones, and it is recommended to perform a cholecystectomy during the exploratory laparotomy. Wedge resection or lobectomy can be performed in some patients with hepatic metastases. Radiofrequency ablation is also used.

Prognosis

There has been hardly any change in the prognosis of endocrine tumors of the small intestine over the past 30 years. The overall 5-year survival rate for endocrine tumors of the small bowel still varies from 52-77%. Some poor prognostic indicators include tumors of larger size, metastases to the lymph nodes, metastases to the liver, carcinoid syndrome, and levels of plasma chromogranin A greater than 5000 mg/ml. The following histologic features also predict poor prognosis: increased invasion depth, vascular/lymphatic involvement, atypical cells, high mitotic index, and necrosis.

Mesenteric Ischemia

Mesenteric ischemia is a result of inadequate blood flow through the mesenteric circulations, which in turn causes ischemia and even gangrene of the wall of the intestine and may be classified as either arterial or venous. Arterial mesenteric ischemia is further grouped into non-occlusive mesenteric ischemia (NOMI) and occlusive mesenteric ischemia (OMAI). OMAI is further grouped into acute mesenteric embolus (AMAE) and acute mesenteric thrombosis (AMAT). Venous mesenteric ischemia is due to mesenteric venous thrombosis (MVT). Mesenteric ischemia may also be due to mechanical obstruction such as a strangulated hernia, volvulus, intussusception, tumor compression, and aortic dissection.

Anatomy

The celiac artery provides vascular supply to the foregut, hepatobiliary system, and spleen. The superior mesenteric artery provides the vascular supply to the small bowel and the proximal mid-colon, while the inferior mesenteric artery provides vascular supply to the distal colon and the rectum. Acute mesenteric ischemia typically is the result of impaired superior mesenteric artery circulation or its venous outflow. The venous outflow is via the superior mesenteric vein, which coalesces with the splenic vein to make the portal vein. The inferior mesenteric artery is rarely the site of an embolus because it has a small luminal diameter.

Pathophysiology

Inadequate perfusion of the small intestine and the colon may be due to occlusion of an artery by an embolus or by a thrombosis, venous thrombosis, vasospasm, or low cardiac output. Embolic events make up 50% of all cases of mesenteric ischemia. Arterial thrombi make up 25%, non-occlusive events make up 20% of all cases of mesenteric ischemia, and mesenteric vein thrombosis accounts for 10% of all cases. The typical pathologic process in mesenteric ischemia is hemorrhagic infarction that results in perforation, whether the occlusion is of arterial or of venous origin.

The degree of injury is inversely proportional to the mesenteric blood flow and depends upon the number of involved blood vessels, the mean systemic blood pressure, the length of time of the ischemic event, and the adequacy of collateral circulation. The superior mesenteric vessels are more commonly involved than the inferior mesenteric vessels because the inferior mesenteric vessels have a better collateral system. Injury seen in mesenteric ischemia may run the gamut from reversible ischemia to bowel wall infarction with necrosis and subsequent perforation. The damage is further complicated by reactive vasospasm.

After the Initial Occlusion

After the initial occlusion, arterial insufficiency results in tissue hypoxia, which causes intestinal wall spasm that results in emptying of the bowel by either vomiting or diarrhea. If the mucosa starts to slough, GI bleeding may be exhibited. Persistent ischemia injures the mucosal barrier and results in bacteria, toxins, and vasoactive materials being discharged into the systemic circulation. Such a discharge of materials may lead to death as a result of septic shock, cardiac failure, or multi-system organ failure prior to the onset of intestinal necrosis. Necrosis of the bowel usually happens 8-12 hours after symptom onset.

Types

Embolic and Thrombotic: Most episodes of embolic acute mesenteric ischemia are secondary to emboli of cardiac origin. Common cardiac causes include mural thrombi status-post myocardial infarction, atrial thrombi as a result of mitral stenosis and atrial fibrillation, vegetative endocarditis, mycotic aneurysm, or plaque thrombi due to atherosclerosis within the aorta or at the location of aortic prosthetic grafts situated anywhere between the heart and the origin of the superior mesenteric artery. The occlusion secondary to an embolus is commonly very sudden in nature; therefore, embolic occlusions will tend to cause more severe ischemia than thrombotic occlusions.

Non-Occlusive: Non-occlusive mesenteric ischemia is commonly secondary to a drastic decrease in mesenteric perfusion and the resultant arterial spasm. Typical causes of non-occlusive mesenteric ischemia include cardiac failure, septic shock, hypovolemia, or the utilization of extreme vasopressors in patients with critical illnesses. The perfusion of the intestine, like that of the perfusion of the brain, is maintained in hypotensive states; thus, non-occlusive mesenteric ischemia is a failure of auto-regulatory mechanisms. Regional vasoconstriction may result in non-occlusive mesenteric ischemia. Vasoactive drugs (digitalis, diuretics, cocaine, and vasopressin are examples) may result in regional vasoconstriction.

VENOUS THROMBOSIS: In more than 80% of cases of mesenteric venous thrombosis the cause is secondary mesenteric venous thrombosis, meaning that the patient has an issue that causes susceptibility to form clots. Primary mesenteric venous thrombosis has no identified cause or predisposing issue. Mesenteric venous thrombosis may also be secondary to extreme surgery for penetrating abdominal trauma; it may also be due to pancreatitis, sickle cell anemia, and malignancy with hypercoagulability.

Etiologies

Etiologies of embolic mesenteric ischemia include cardiac emboli, plaque emboli derived from atherosclerotic areas, and plaque dislodged during heart catheterization. Thrombotic mesenteric ischemia: atherosclerotic vascular disease (most common cause), aortic aneurysm, aortic dissection, arteritis, acute cardiac decompensation from AMAT with concomitant reduced cardiac output as a result of AMI or CHF, and dehydration. Non-occlusive mesenteric ischemia: hypotension secondary to CHF, myocardial infarction, sepsis, AI, severe hepatic/renal disease, vasopressors, ergotamines, cocaine, and digitalis. Mesenteric venous thrombosis: hypercoagulability from protein S and protein C deficiency, antithrombin-III deficiency, dysfibrinogenemia, polycythemia vera, oral contraceptives, and pregnancy, tumor-compression or paraneoplastic syndrome, infection, portal hypertension, venous trauma, pancreatitis, and decompression illness.

Epidemiology and Prognosis

Acute mesenteric ischemia has a prevalence of 0.1% of all hospital admissions in the United States. Rates of acute mesenteric ischemia are lower outside of the United States secondary to limited diagnostic methods and lower life expectancy. Acute mesenteric ischemia usually occurs in patients over age 50 but may occur in younger patients with atrial fibrillation or risk factors for mesenteric venous thrombosis. There is no overall gender difference or racial predilection for acute mesenteric ischemia. Any type of acute mesenteric ischemia has a poor prognosis. The overall mortality due to all causes averages 71%.

GI Symptoms in Addison's Disease

Addison's disease is also known as adrenal insufficiency. Adrenal insufficiency may be precipitated by infection or stress and result in an acute crisis that is characterized by hypotension, hypovolemic shock, acute abdominal pain, fever, and vomiting. Adrenal insufficiency may also be manifested by chronic symptoms of fatigue, hyper-pigmentation, weight loss, anorexia or appetite loss, early satiety, nausea and vomiting, abdominal pain (may present like an acute abdomen), and unusual cravings for soy sauce, salt, or licorice. An acute adrenal crisis may be misdiagnosed as acute gastroenteritis because nausea and vomiting are key symptoms.

Review Video: Addison's Disease
Visit mometrix.com/academy and enter code: 813552

GI Symptoms in Thyroid Disease

The GI manifestations of thyroid disease are numerous. Motor dysfunction of the GI tract is thought to be the primary cause of GI symptoms in thyroid disease and exhibits alterations in bowel motility and in transit time. GI symptoms in hyperthyroidism occur in 30-50% of patients. GI symptoms in hyperthyroidism may include increased frequency of bowel movements, diarrhea, and malabsorption with steatorrhea. Other symptoms that are often noted include dyspepsia, epigastric pain, early satiety, belching, nausea, and vomiting. Rare cases of intractable vomiting have been noted in patients with hyperthyroidism.

Skin Findings in Small Bowel Disease

Peutz-Jeghers syndrome is autosomal dominant and demonstrates mucocutaneous hyperpigmentation and GI polyposis. Skin lesions are bluish-brown in nature and macular. The most common location is the lips. GI manifestations of Peutz-Jeghers syndrome are numerous hamartomatous polyps that are most typically noted in the jejunum but may also be noted in the stomach, duodenum, ileum, and colon. Such polyps may cause abdominal pain, GI bleeding, rectal prolapse, and obstruction secondary to intussusception. There is also a 2-3% chance of developing a GI carcinoma with this disorder. Upper and lower endoscopy is suggested every 2 years in these patients.

Skin Lesions and GI Symptoms in HSP

HSP (Henoch-Schönlein purpura) is a vasculitis of small vessels that exhibits palpable purpura, arthralgias, abdominal symptoms, and glomerulonephritis. Most of the lesions are found on the buttocks and the legs. 50% of patients with HSP will have GI symptoms. The GI symptoms of HSP include abdominal pain that is colicky in nature, diarrhea or constipation, occult/overt GI bleeding, intussusception, and perforation. GI findings of HSP on endoscopy are extreme diffuse erythema, raised lesions, numerous areas of ulceration, and diffuse erosions. With HSP, the duodenum and the small bowel are the most common sites for involvement.

Colon

Anorectal Disease

Anorectal disease may be present in any patient with HIV infection but is more likely in homosexual men. There is an increased frequency of anorectal disease in homosexual men with advanced HIV infection. Common presentations of anorectal disease may include perirectal abscesses, anal fistulae, infectious proctitis, lymphoma, ulcerations secondary to tuberculosis, and histoplasmosis. Nonspecific ulcerations may also be seen and are like those seen in esophagitis. Anorectal carcinoma is more prevalent in the homosexual male population; such carcinoma is thought to be secondary to chronic perianal HSV or papillomavirus. Patients with HIV infection who are not homosexual males do not have a high prevalence of anorectal carcinoma.

Diverticulitis

Diverticula are defined as "small mucosal herniations protruding through the intestinal layers and the smooth muscle along the natural openings created by the vasa recta or nutrient vessels in the wall of the colon." Such herniations result in small pouches that are lined solely with mucosa and may occur anywhere in the GI tract but are most typically found in the colon. Diverticulitis is defined as "an inflammation of one or more diverticula." A diverticulum may become obstructed, which leads to distention, impaired vascularity, and micro- or macroperforation. One of the complications of diverticulitis is fistula formation.

Epidemiology

Diverticulitis is more frequent in patients with large numbers of diverticula: 15-20% of patients with diverticulosis develop diverticulitis; 20% of patients with diverticulitis are younger than 50 years. Most patients with diverticulosis do not have symptoms (80-85%); 5% have diverticulitis; and 15-20% develops complications that necessitate surgery. Complications that require surgery include abscess, intestinal rupture, formation of fistulae, and peritonitis. Race is a factor, with left-sided diverticulitis seen in the United States and right-sided diverticulitis seen in Asians. The rate of diverticulitis is similar between men and women.

Clinical Presentation

The presenting symptoms of diverticulitis will depend upon the location of disease. LLQ pain is the most typical symptom and occurs in 70% of patients. Some other symptoms include nausea, cramping, change in bowel habits, vomiting, constipation, diarrhea, flatulence, and bloating. Diverticulitis may develop in any portion of the GI tract; therefore, it can mimic other diseases. Examples of diverticulitis mimicking other disease include right-sided diverticulitis acting like appendicitis; transverse colon diverticulitis acting like pancreatitis, peptic ulcer, or cholecystitis; retroperitoneal diverticulitis acting like kidney or renal disease; and lower quadrant pain in women acting like gynecological disease.

The symptoms of severe diverticulitis may include anorexia, nausea, vomiting, localized pain (usually severe), alterations in bowel habits (usually constipation), and even urinary symptoms of dysuria, urgency, and increased frequency (due to irritation of nearby urinary structures). Macroperforation will result in generalized abdominal pain and peritonitis. Rare instances of leg pain associated with emphysematous changes have been reported as a consequence of retroperitoneal diverticular perforation. In a simple case of diverticulitis, fever and localized pain may be present. Abscess formation as a resultant complication may be detected as a tender mass.

Differential Diagnosis

The differential diagnosis of diverticulitis is extensive and includes appendicitis, biliary colic, biliary disease, biliary obstruction, cholangitis, cholecystitis, chronic mesenteric ischemia, obstruction of the colon, fistula between the colon and the bladder, constipation, duodenal ulcer, gastric ulcer, acute gastritis, viral gastroenteritis, pain from gynecological diseases, inflammatory bowel disease, perforation of the intestine, sepsis secondary to an intra-abdominal process, irritable bowel syndrome, hepatic abscess, ischemia of the mesenteric artery, thrombosis of the mesenteric artery, kidney stones, acute renal colic, ovarian cyst, acute pancreatitis, pelvic inflammatory disease, acute pyelonephritis, rectovaginal fistula, and urinary tract infection or obstruction.

Lab Work-Up

Diverticulitis is most often diagnosed on the basis of the history and physical. Laboratory studies are sometimes needed, however. CBC may show an elevated WBC count with a left shift, but 20-40% of patients with diverticulitis do not exhibit a high WBC count with a left shift, especially patients with immunocompromise and the elderly. Electrolytes are indicated in patient who presents with vomiting and diarrhea; creatinine should be assessed prior to IV contrast administration. UA and urine culture may be helpful in distinguishing between UTI and sterile pyuria from inflammation of nearby urinary structures.

Imaging Studies

The gold standard in using imaging studies in the diagnosis of diverticulitis is the CT of the abdomen. CT of the abdomen is considered to be safer than contrast studies in the acute setting and may also allow an assessment of the severity of the diverticular disease, any complications that may be concurrent, and clinical staging. Some findings on CT of the abdomen may include inflammatory changes of pericolic fat stranding, diverticula in the colon, thickening of the wall of the bowel, inflammatory masses located in soft tissue, phlegmon, and the presence of abscesses.

Clinical Staging

Many forms of staging methods have been suggested for the clinical staging of diverticulitis and have been based upon clinical findings, the extent of disease on imaging studies, and the presence of complications. Some physicians recommend clinical staging based upon the differentiation between asymptomatic diverticulosis, uncomplicated diverticulitis, and complicated diverticulitis. Hinchey's classification of clinical staging is typically utilized as a means of selecting the appropriate surgical procedure for the treatment of complicated diverticulitis. Stage I disease is considered to be a small or confined pericolic or mesenteric abscess; Stage II disease is a large abscess that is often confined to the pelvis; Stage III is perforation causing suppurative peritonitis; and Stage IV is rupture with fecal contamination and generalized fecal peritonitis.

Medical Management and Treatment

Acute uncomplicated diverticulitis may be treated and managed medically in 70-100% of patients. Often, the presence of mild diverticulitis may be treated with an outpatient plan that is comprised of a clear liquid diet and an appropriate course of antibiotics. Antibiotics will need to cover anaerobes (*B. fragilis*, *Peptostreptococcus*, *Clostridium*) and aerobes (*E. Coli*, *Klebsiella*, *Proteus*, etc.), a typical regimen is a combination of ciprofloxacin or co-trimoxazole and metronidazole. Moxifloxacin and amoxicillin/clavulanate are also antibiotic treatments for uncomplicated and simple diverticulitis. Hospitalization may be indicated for severe diverticulitis or in patients with severe dehydration, etc.

Surgical Indications

In patients presenting with a primary episode of acute diverticulitis, 15-25% will need surgery secondary to complications; 15-30% of patients admitted for management of acute diverticulitis will require surgery with an 18% mortality rate (WGO, 2007). The classic surgical indications for diverticulitis are "free-air perforation with fecal perforation, suppurative peritonitis secondary to a ruptured abscess, uncontrolled sepsis, abdominal or pelvic abscess (unless CT-guided aspiration is possible), fistula formation, inability to rule out carcinoma, intestinal obstruction, failing medical therapy, immunocompromised status, and extremes of age." Preoperative administration of antibiotics is a usual practice.

Endocrine Tumors of the Colon

Endocrine tumors of the colon are quite rare and account for only 1% of all colon cancers. Most patients are in the 65-70-year age group. Two-thirds of patients will have tumors that are greater than 5 cm in diameter and will have local or distant metastases. The overall 5-year survival rate is from 25-41% in these patients. The most common symptoms in patients with colon or rectal endocrine tumors are anorexia, abdominal pain, and unintentional weight loss. Rectal endocrine tumors are usually asymptomatic and are often found upon examination.

Rectal Endocrine Tumors

Most rectal endocrine tumors are not symptomatic but symptoms may include rectal bleeding, rectal pain, or constipation. Endocrine tumors of the rectum make up only 1.3% of all rectal neoplasms. Endocrine tumors of the rectum are derived from epithelial endocrine cells and typically contain glucagon and glicentin-like peptides as opposed to serotonin. Carcinoid syndrome is quite rare in endocrine tumors of the rectum. If the endocrine tumor of the rectum is smaller than 1 cm in diameter, metastasis is unusual; however, if the primary tumor is larger than 2 cm, metastasis will be seen in 70% of cases.

Radiation Proctitis

Radiation proctitis is also known as post-radiation telangiectasia and is the formation of telangiectasia after radiation treatment to the floor of the pelvis (usually for cervical or prostate cancer). Such lesions typically appear a few months after radiation therapy, but some patients have had radiation proctitis as late as 2 years after radiation treatments. The histologic findings include fibrosis of the connective tissue, obliterative endarteritis, and neovascularization secondary to chronic ischemia. Treatment is somewhat difficult but can include formalin rectal enemas, topical steroids, sucralfate enemas, and 5-aminosalicylate preparations. Currently, argon plasma coagulation (APC) via endoscopy is widely used.

GI Manifestations of Rheumatoid Arthritis

Many systemic diseases have GI manifestations. Rheumatoid arthritis has been associated with both upper and lower GI symptoms. Most of the upper GI symptoms that are associated with rheumatoid arthritis are secondary to medications—especially nonsteroidal anti-inflammatory drugs. There has been a 50% increase in the incidence of lower GI problems in patients with rheumatoid arthritis. Risk factors for lower GI problems in these patients include smoking, steroid administration, previous upper GI disease, and previous abdominal surgery. Upper GI issues in RA include GI bleed, GI perforation, ulcer, obstruction, and esophagitis. Lower GI issues in RA patients include bleeding, perforation, ulcers, obstruction, diverticulitis, and colitis.

GI Manifestations of Lupus

GI manifestations of systemic lupus may be primary disorders such as gastritis, peptic ulcer, pancreatitis, and biliary disease. Some of the GI manifestations, however, are secondary to the disease itself. Lupus-associated GI issues may include small and large intestinal ischemia due to vasculitis or occlusion from anti-phospholipid syndrome or peritonitis from serositis. Vasculitis involving the intestine is thought to occur in 2% of patients with systemic lupus and delay in diagnosis may result in bowel infarction and perforation. The vasculitis seen in systemic lupus may occur anywhere in the GI tract.

GI Symptoms in Paraneoplastic Syndromes

Paraneoplastic syndromes are "rare disorders that are triggered by an altered immune system response to a neoplasm." Symptoms from paraneoplastic syndromes may be endocrine, musculoskeletal, cardiac, cutaneous, hematologic, GI, neurologic, and renal in nature. Fever is the most common presenting symptom but these syndromes may run the gamut from dermatomyositis-polymyositis to Cushing syndrome to malignant carcinoid syndrome. Some of the GI symptoms of paraneoplastic syndromes include watery diarrhea (which causes electrolyte issues that result in weakness, confusion, and exhaustion), malabsorption (typically noted with proctosigmoid tumors and medullary thyroid carcinomas), and malnutrition due to malabsorption.

Inflammatory Bowel Disease

There are two forms of inflammatory bowel disease, Crohn disease and ulcerative colitis. The cause of inflammatory bowel disease is not clear but is thought to be due to an immune reaction of the patient to his own intestinal tract. Ulcerative colitis is limited to the colon while Crohn disease may involve the GI tract in its entirety and have lesions from the mouth to the anus. Ulcerative colitis always has rectal involvement. There is a genetic pre-disposition to both forms of inflammatory bowel disease with an increased tendency to develop malignant neoplastic lesions.

Both forms of inflammatory bowel disease exhibit extra-intestinal manifestations. Systemic symptoms such as fever, sweats, arthralgias, and malaise are also common to both diseases. The lesions found in ulcerative colitis are continuous and involve both the mucosa and the submucosa. The lesions in Crohn disease are "skip" lesions and are transmural in nature. The symptoms of both ulcerative colitis and Crohn disease may wax and wane in intensity and in severity. Many of the patients with ulcerative colitis or Crohn disease may have concomitant irritable bowel syndrome; therefore, medications should be used with caution.

Etiologies

There are several factors that have been suggested that may be the initiating event for the immune response activation seen in inflammatory bowel disease. These factors include a pathogenic organism, the presence of an intraluminal antigen that causes an immune response, or an autoimmune response to an impairment in barrier function. The immune response activation seen in inflammatory bowel disease is polyclonal in that acute neutrophilic and chronic lymphocytic aspects are noted. There is a genetic predisposition in inflammatory bowel disease; 10-25% of patients with inflammatory bowel disease also have a first-degree family member with the disease.

Epidemiology

Approximately 2 million people in the United States have either ulcerative colitis or Crohn disease. The rate of incidence is 70-150 cases per 100,000. The prevalence of inflammatory bowel disease in African Americans is the same as in Americans of European descent; however, the prevalence is less in Asian Americans and in Hispanic Americans. Caucasians have a fourfold higher incidence of inflammatory bowel disease, with the greatest rates noted in the Jewish population. American Jews have a four- to five-fold greater prevalence of inflammatory bowel disease. The male-to-female ratio is about equal for both forms of inflammatory bowel disease.

Clinical Presentation

The clinical presentation of inflammatory bowel disease will depend upon the location of the lesions. Some patients with inflammatory bowel disease will also have irritable bowel syndrome and will exhibit symptoms of cramping, irregular bowel habits, and mucus (typically without the presence of blood or pus). Frequent systemic symptoms are noted and include fever, sweats, malaise, and arthralgias. Fatigue is a common symptom and may be secondary to anemia, pain, and inflammation that go along with the disease. Flares may be due to stress, infection, acute illness, pregnancy, diet, and various medications. Grossly bloody stools are more commonly seen in ulcerative colitis than in Crohn disease, with loose bowel movements being the norm if there is extensive involvement of the colon or the terminal ileum. 50% of patients with Crohn disease will exhibit perianal disease such as fistulas or abscesses. Numerous intestinal and extra-intestinal issues may be present in both forms of inflammatory bowel disease. Significant weight loss is more commonly noted in Crohn disease than in ulcerative colitis secondary to small bowel malabsorption. Patients may decrease their food intake as a means of trying to alleviate symptoms.

Ulcerative Colitis

The common pathologic pathway in both forms of inflammatory bowel disease is inflammation of the lining of the GI tract that results in ulceration, edema, bleeding, and fluid/electrolyte losses. In ulcerative colitis, the inflammatory process originates in the rectum and goes in a proximal fashion to eventually cause involvement in the entire large intestine. The lesions are continuous, unlike in Crohn disease, and are confined to the rectum alone in 25% of patients. 75% of patients with ulcerative colitis have lesions that extend in a proximal manner and involve the entire large bowel. Ulcerative colitis is considered to be surgically curable. Indications for colectomy in ulcerative colitis include difficulty in managing inflammation and potential malignant changes noted upon surveillance (such as high-grade dysplasia, presence of strictures, intolerance of medication side effects, and poor quality of life secondary to the disease). There are 2 common surgical treatments for ulcerative colitis: proctocolectomy with ileostomy and total colectomy with ileoanal anastomosis. Total proctocolectomy with creation of an ileostomy is thought to be the easier procedure and has the lowest complication rates.

Crohn Disease

Crohn disease may involve any element of the GI tract from the mouth to the anus and exhibits 3 distinct patterns of involvement: inflammatory, strictures, and fistulas. Crohn disease is characterized by segmental areas of an inflammatory granulomatous process that is not specific in nature. An important distinguishing feature of Crohn disease is the fact that it is a transmural process in that it affects all the layers of the bowel wall. Ulcerative colitis affects the mucosa and the submucosa. 40% of patients with Crohn disease have lesions in the ileum and the cecum, 30% have lesions only in the small bowel, and 25% have lesions only in the colon.

Rectal sparing is commonly seen in Crohn disease but is not thought to be a constant aspect of the disease. Fistulas and abscesses in the anorectal area, however, are often seen in Crohn disease. Sometimes Crohn disease may be exhibited in the proximal GI tract with lesions in the mouth, tongue, esophagus, stomach, and duodenum. Crohn disease has a high incidence of gallstones and kidney stones as a result of malabsorption of fat and of bile salts. Increased gallstone formation is secondary to an increased cholesterol concentration in bile due to a decreased bile salt concentration.

Most surgical treatment used in Crohn disease is to manage complications such as fistula, stricture, or bleeding; 50% of patients with Crohn disease will need some form of surgical intervention. The rate of recurrence after surgery is very high—100% of those patients needing surgery will have a recurrence within 1 year. After surgery, the recurrence typically mimics the original pattern of disease, with the recurrence being noted on one or both aspects of the anastomosis. Surgical procedures utilized with Crohn disease may include segmental resection, bowel-sparing stricturoplasty, and diverting ileostomy or colostomy.

Differences in the Presentation of Ulcerative Colitis and Crohn Disease

There are distinguishing features to be noted between the clinical presentation of ulcerative colitis and of Crohn disease. "Skip" areas are frequently seen in Crohn disease but are never seen in ulcerative colitis. A cobblestone mucosa is commonly seen in Crohn disease but is rarely noted in ulcerative colitis. Transmural bowel involvement is typical of Crohn disease but is rarely noted in ulcerative colitis. Sparing of the rectum often occurs in Crohn disease but is never noted in ulcerative colitis. Perianal issues are common in Crohn disease but never occur in ulcerative colitis.

Complications

20% of patients with inflammatory bowel disease will have extra-intestinal issues. Intestinal complications associated with inflammatory bowel disease can include fistulas, strictures, abscesses, perforation, toxic megacolon, and neoplasm. Extra-intestinal manifestations of inflammatory bowel disease include osteoporosis, hypercoagulable states, anemia, gallstones, primary sclerosing cholangitis, aphthous ulcers, iritis, uveitis, episcleritis, pyoderma gangrenosum, and erythema nodosum. The following are more commonly seen in Crohn disease than in ulcerative colitis: arthritis, aphthous stomatitis, uveitis, erythema nodosum, ankylosing spondylitis, and psoriasis. Pyoderma gangrenosum is seen with equal prevalence in Crohn disease and in ulcerative colitis, while sclerosing cholangitis is more commonly seen with ulcerative colitis.

Differential Diagnosis

Numerous conditions may present in a similar manner to inflammatory bowel disease. Such conditions may include AIDS with Kaposi sarcoma that involves the intestine, antibiotic-associated colitis, AV malformations, backwash ileitis, C1 esterase deficiency, infectious colitis, intestinal lymphoma, intestinal tuberculosis, irritable bowel syndrome, ischemic colitis, pseudomembranous colitis, radiation-induced colitis, chronic schistosomiasis and amebiasis, chronic Yersinia infection, lymphogranuloma venereum, actinomycosis, chronic diverticulitis, Behçet syndrome, NSAID-enteropathy, anorexia nervosa, appendicitis, celiac sprue, *C. difficile* colitis, CMV infection and CMV colitis, food poisoning, bacterial and viral gastroenteritis, giardiasis, disorders of intestinal motility, radiation injury to the intestine, lactose intolerance, and *Salmonella* infection.

Laboratory and Stool Studies

A CBC is useful in the diagnosis of inflammatory bowel disease because it may serve as an indicator of disease activity and of iron and vitamin deficiencies. A high WBC count is typically noted but usually represents inflammation as opposed to infection. Anemia is frequently noted on CBC and may be anemia of chronic disease or iron-deficiency anemia; the anemia noted may also be secondary to blood loss or malabsorption. ESR is often utilized as a general marker for inflammation and disease activity. Stool studies are often used to rule out infectious processes.

X-Ray Studies

Flat-plate and upright abdomen films can be useful in the diagnosis of inflammatory bowel disease. Findings may include a colon that appears irregular and edematous with "thumb-printing." Free air and air in the wall of the colon may be noted, as well as the presence of toxic megacolon. Other findings may be signs of kidney stones, gallstones, and arthritis. Barium enema may show a "lead-pipe" appearance in ulcerative colitis, rectal sparing that is associated with Crohn disease, "thumb-printing" that indicates mucosal involvement, or "skip lesions" that are associated with Crohn disease.

Colonoscopy

Colonoscopy can be an extremely useful tool in the diagnosis of inflammatory bowel disease. However, it is important to consider the infectious causes of inflammation, as well as ischemic colitis and diverticulitis. Colonoscopy is useful in delineating the severity and the extent of disease, directing treatment options, and obtaining tissue samples. The rectum will always be involved in ulcerative colitis, while a right-sided colonic predominance is usually noted with Crohn disease. Ulcerative colitis may be noted in the rectum only; the rectum, sigmoid, and descending colon; or the entire colon. It is not seen in any other aspect of the GI tract.

Symptomatic Treatment

Treatment of inflammatory bowel disease may require a combination of both medical and surgical therapies. Symptomatic treatment may include agents to control diarrhea, bind bile acids, prevent spasm, and suppress acid production. Loperamide in combination with diphenoxylate and atropine has been used to decrease the number of bowel movements and to alleviate rectal urgency. Cholestyramine is a bile salt binding agent that may be needed to decrease diarrhea in patients with Crohn disease who have had an ileal resection. It is vital to recall that antidiarrheal and anticholinergic medications may cause toxic megacolon.

Stepwise Therapy

Aminosalicylates are typically the first step in medication treatment for inflammatory bowel disease. The next step is the use of corticosteroids that have the advantage of providing fast relief from symptoms and reducing inflammation. The typical dose of oral prednisone is 10-40 mg per day with a taper that is initiated once clinical improvement in symptoms is seen. Step 3 medications include immune modifying agents or tumor necrosis factor (TNF). Step 3 medications are typically utilized if steroids fail or are needed for long periods of time. Step 4 medications are experimental agents.

Immune-Modifying Medications

Immune-modifying medications that are used in treating inflammatory bowel disease include 6-MP and azathioprine. These medications function to decrease the lymphocyte count and usually take 2-3 months to achieve effective onset of action. Such medications are often needed in light of their steroid-sparing action in patients that suffer refractory disease and are also used as a primary treatment for fistula and to maintain remission in patients who cannot tolerate the aminosalicylates. It is critical to closely monitor CBC and LFTs because immune modifying medications may cause dramatic neutropenia and/or pancytopenia.

Extra-Intestinal Manifestations: Approximately 25-40% of patients with inflammatory bowel disease will have extra-intestinal manifestations. One large study demonstrated that extra-intestinal manifestations are more likely in patients with Crohn disease than in patients with ulcerative colitis. Such manifestations are linked to active inflammatory bowel disease in over 90% of patients. Extra-intestinal manifestations parallel disease activity in the following conditions: peripheral arthritis (large joint involvement is greater than small joint involvement), erythema nodosum, pyoderma gangrenosum, and episcleritis. Extra-intestinal manifestations that do not parallel disease activity are primary sclerosing cholangitis, uveitis, and axial arthropathy.

Peripheral Arthropathy

Approximately 5-20% of patients with inflammatory bowel disease exhibit signs of peripheral arthropathy. Patients with Crohn disease have a greater incidence of peripheral arthropathy than patients with ulcerative colitis. Peripheral arthropathy is more likely in patients with Crohn disease with involvement of the colon and in ulcerative colitis patients who have extensive colonic disease. There is a greater risk of peripheral arthropathy if complications of inflammatory bowel disease and extra-intestinal manifestations are present. There is typically no permanent deformity of the joints noted; the peripheral arthropathy will commonly respond to treatment of the inflammatory bowel disease.

Axial Arthropathy

Axial arthropathy as an extra-intestinal manifestation of inflammatory bowel disease is less likely than peripheral arthropathy, with only 3-5% of patients exhibiting such symptoms. Axial arthropathy is manifested as sacroiliitis and spondylitis and is characterized by low back pain and early morning stiffness. The symptoms of axial arthropathy do not parallel disease activity. 5-10% of patients with axial arthropathy will have signs and symptoms of spondylitis; most patients are HLA-B27 positive. Spondylitis typically is progressive and causes permanent damage to the spine. Most patients with sacroiliitis do not have symptoms, are HLA-B27 negative, and usually do not progress to spondylitis.

Osteopenia and Osteoporosis

In patients with Crohn disease, 30-60% will have signs and symptoms of osteopenia and/or osteoporosis secondary to the poor absorption of calcium and vitamin D as well as the result of inflammatory action of cytokines and osteoblasts. Chronic steroid administration exacerbates osteoporosis in these patients. There is a higher risk of osteoporosis and osteopenia in patients with Crohn disease even in the presence of a normal body mass density. All patients over age 60 with inflammatory bowel disease or women who are post-menopausal are recommended to undergo DEXA screening.

Pyoderma Gangrenosum

Pyoderma gangrenosum is noted in about 5% of patients with ulcerative colitis and is much less commonly seen in patients with Crohn disease. The most common locations for the lesions of pyoderma gangrenosum are the leg or surrounding a stoma, though they may also be seen on the face, trunk, or upper limbs. Pathergy is a characteristic of pyoderma gangrenosum and means that the lesions will get worse with trauma or debridement. Lesions typically start as a papules, pustules, or nodules, and then go on to ulcerate and parallel disease activity in ulcerative colitis but not in Crohn disease.

Ocular Manifestations

About 10% of patients with inflammatory bowel disease will exhibit ocular manifestations. Ocular manifestations in inflammatory bowel disease may cause permanent vision loss. An urgent referral to an ophthalmologist is typically necessary for scleritis and uveitis. Signs and symptoms of ocular manifestations include tearing, burning, itching, eye pain, photophobia, hyperemia of the conjunctiva or sclera, blurry vision, and loss of visual acuity. Episcleritis presents as acute onset of redness in one or in both eyes with irritation and burning. Pain is a typical symptom; episcleritis will flare with a disease flare and improve with treatment of the inflammatory bowel disease.

Scleritis and Uveitis

Scleritis is generally more severe in nature than episcleritis and causes severe ocular pain with extensive and diffuse erythema noted. Complications of scleritis may include vision loss, detachment of the retina, and swelling of the optic nerve. Scleritis typically necessitates urgent referral and is treated with nonsteroidal antiinflammatory drugs, systemic steroids, or immunosuppressants in order to prevent loss of vision. Uveitis is characterized by ocular pain, blurry vision, and photophobia, and demonstrates signs of "ciliary flush." Complications of uveitis include intraocular adhesions that may ultimately result in cataracts and glaucoma.

Primary Sclerosing Cholangitis

Primary sclerosing cholangitis (PSC) is the most common hepatobiliary complication seen in inflammatory bowel disease; 70-80% of patients with PSC have inflammatory bowel disease as well. There is a distinct pattern of clinical findings in patients with PSC and inflammatory bowel disease: "higher prevalence of rectal sparing, more backwash ileitis, more likely to have pancolitis, higher incidence of colorectal neoplasia, and poorer survival overall." PSC is noted in 85-90% of patients with ulcerative colitis as opposed to 7.5% of patients with Crohn disease. The course of PSC is independent of the course of the inflammatory bowel disease.

Pancreatitis and Gallstones

Acute and chronic pancreatitis may be seen in patients with inflammatory bowel disease since these patients have a greater risk secondary to gallstones, medications (5-ASA, Imuran, steroids, and 6-MP), or simply idiopathic causes. Most patients do not have symptoms. The risk is slightly elevated for patients with Crohn disease as opposed to ulcerative colitis. 17-34% of patients with Crohn disease will have gallstones as a result of a decreased bile salt pool, which is secondary to decreased terminal ileal resorption. Decreased bile salt pool results in cholesterol supersaturation and gallstone formation.

Kidney Stones

Kidney stones occur in 7-10% of patients with inflammatory bowel disease and are usually composed of uric acid or calcium oxalate. Calcium oxalate stones account for 80% of kidney stones in patients with inflammatory bowel disease because of malabsorption of fat, which results in binding of fatty acids to calcium, and subsequently less calcium to bind with and to clear oxalate. It is important to note that calcium oxalate stones will only occur with an intact colon. Uric acid stones result from volume depletion and an increased metabolic state and are typically noted in patients with an ileostomy.

Colorectal Cancer

Inflammatory bowel disease is associated with an increased risk of colorectal cancer secondary to the presence of longstanding inflammation. Risk factors include the duration and the extent of inflammatory bowel disease, the presence of severe inflammation upon endoscopy, primary sclerosing cholangitis, a positive family history of colon cancer, and a younger age at time of diagnosis. Inflammatory bowel disease also exhibits a greater risk of developing other intestinal cancers such as lymphoma, small bowel adenocarcinoma, pouch neoplasia, and perianal neoplasia. Studies note that the risk of colorectal cancer is substantial after 10 years with inflammatory bowel disease.

Surveillance Guidelines

The following have been suggested as screening surveillance guidelines for patients with inflammatory bowel disease: initial screening colonoscopy for patients with ulcerative colitis and extensive or left-sided colitis and in patients with Crohn disease that involves at least one-third of the colon. Screening is recommended at 8-10 years after the onset of extensive ulcerative colitis or in patients with Crohn colitis, which affects more than 50% of the colon. A screening colonoscopy is suggested at 15 years after disease onset for left-sided ulcerative colitis or Crohn colitis involving more than one-third of the colon.

C. Difficile Colitis

C. difficile is a gram-positive, anaerobic, spore-forming bacillus that is the etiologic agent in antibiotic-associated diarrhea and colitis. Infection with *C. difficile* presents with mild to moderate diarrhea and abdominal cramping. Pseudomembranes, which are plaques present on the mucosa of the intestine, may be seen on occasion. 20% of hospitalized patients will acquire *C. difficile*, 30% of these patients will have diarrhea. *C. difficile* is thought to be one of the most common nosocomial infections. *C. difficile* should be considered in the following patients: diarrhea if antibiotics have been given in the prior 2 months and diarrhea starting within 72 hours of hospitalization.

Pathophysiology

"C. difficile colitis results from a disturbance of the normal bacterial flora of the colon, colonization with *C. difficile*, and release of toxins that cause mucosal inflammation and damage." Antibiotic treatment is the primary cause of alteration in colonic flora. Hospitalized patients are at greater risk of *C. difficile* infection; transmission is via a fecal-oral route. The normal flora of the colon prevents colonization with *C. difficile* and also prevents overgrowth of *C. difficile. C. difficile* makes two toxins: Toxin A is an enterotoxin, and toxin B is a cytotoxin. Both toxins contribute to *C. difficile* colitis.

Epidemiology

In the United States, it is estimated that *C. difficile* is the cause of 3 million cases of diarrhea and colitis a year. Most nosocomial infections decreased from 2000-2009 but infections secondary to *C. difficile* rose more than 50%. According to the CDC in 2010, 94% of *C. difficile* infections were a result of health care; 75% of these cases were in patients who were not presently hospitalized—meaning recently discharged patients, outpatients, and residents of nursing homes. Most patients with *C. difficile* infection recover; however, the mortality rate in seriously ill patients ranges from 10-30%.

Clinical Presentation

Colonization with *C. difficile* may range from being an asymptomatic carrier, including mild and self-limited diarrhea and pseudomembranous colitis, to fulminant colitis. Studies demonstrate that up to 25-40% of patients may not exhibit symptoms of *C. difficile* infection for up to 10 weeks after antibiotic treatment. Common symptoms of *C. difficile* infection include mild to moderate watery diarrhea that is occasionally bloody in nature, cramping abdominal pain, anorexia, malaise, and fever. Upon physical examination, the following may be noted: fever, dehydration, lower abdominal pain, and rebound tenderness (increases suspicion of perforation of the colon and peritonitis).

Risk Factors

The primary culprit in *C. difficile* infection is prior antibiotic treatment. The most common antibiotics are second- and third-generation cephalosporins, ampicillin, amoxicillin, and clindamycin. Less common antibiotic causes are erythromycin, clarithromycin, azithromycin, and other forms of penicillin. There have been occasional reports of *C. difficile* colitis secondary to aminoglycosides, fluoroquinolones, co-trimoxazole, metronidazole, chloramphenicol, tetracycline, imipenem, and meropenem. Some other risk factors include age over 60 years and hospitalization—especially sharing a room with an infected patient, ICU stays, and prolonged hospital stays. Other rare factors associated with infection are PPI use, methotrexate, intestinal ischemia, and others.

Differential Diagnosis

The differential diagnosis list for *C. difficile* colitis includes many disorders, such as Crohn disease, diverticulitis, viral gastroenteritis infection, inflammatory bowel disease, sepsis from an intra-abdominal source, irritable bowel syndrome, syndromes of malabsorption and conditions that cause malabsorption, toxic megacolon, pseudomembranous colitis, infection with *Salmonella*, infection with *Shigella*, ulcerative colitis, and infection secondary to vibrio. It is important to perform laboratory studies to assess dehydration and electrolyte depletion, in any case but stool culture is considered to be the most sensitive test for *C. difficile* colitis.

Treatment

Asymptomatic carriers of *C. difficile* do not need treatment. Stopping the offending antibiotic may be the only treatment necessary for mild cases of diarrhea that are not accompanied by fever, abdominal pain, and an elevated WBC count. Patients with moderate diarrhea or *C. difficile* colitis typically require treatment with metronidazole (oral or IV) or vancomycin (oral) for a ten-day course. Vancomycin is thought to be superior to metronidazole in severe cases because of faster resolution of symptoms and a decreased rate of treatment failure.

Relapse

Studies show that relapse will occur in 20-27% of patients with *C. difficile* colitis who have been treated with metronidazole or vancomycin, the risk of another relapse following an initial relapse is 45%. A poor immune response to *C. difficile* and persistent alteration in gut flora increases the risk of relapse. To treat a relapse that occurs after a first relapse, a prolonged vancomycin taper with a pulsed regimen is suggested. IV immunoglobulin (IV Ig) has been studied as an adjunct for treatment of relapsing *C. difficile* colitis as a boost to the poor host immune response.

Colon Cancer

Cancer of the colon is the second leading cause of cancer death in the United States; the lifetime risk for the development of cancer of the colon is 1 in 17. There are multiple environmental and demographic risk factors for cancer of the colon. Environmental factors are noted to be a large etiologic factor in cancer of the colon in spite of the importance of genetic mutations that contribute to the development of cancer of the colon. The industrialized nations have the greatest incidence of cancer of the colon, while South America and China have a low incidence of colon cancer.

Evironmental Risk Factors

There are multiple environmental risk factors for colon cancer. Advanced age is a risk factor; the possible mechanism is the increase in acquired cell mutations. Residing in highly industrialized nations (barring Japan) is thought to increase the risk secondary to dietary and environmental carcinogen exposures. Lack of exercise may decrease immunosurveillance and peristalsis, which results in increased contact of the mucosa with fecal carcinogens. Dietary risk factors have been suggested and include high fat, large amounts of red meat, low amounts of fruit and vegetables, and low levels of selenium, folate, and calcium. Obesity, smoking, and alcohol consumption are also thought to be risk factors.

Family and Genetic Risk Factors

Familial adenomatous polyposis is a genetic condition in which there is the development of multiple small colonic adenomatous polyps that eventually cause cancer of the colon secondary to the risk of malignant transformation inherent in each adenomatous polyp. Lynch syndrome is a variant of familial adenomatous polyposis wherein mutation of a repair gene results in a large number of mutations—especially of tumor suppressor genes. Peutz-Jeghers syndrome exhibits hamartomatous polyps that may become adenomas. Juvenile polyposis exhibits polyps that may become cancerous adenomas. A family history of colon cancer is a risk factor, as well as having hyperplastic polyposis.

Other Possible Risk Factors

Inflammatory bowel disease is a known risk factor for colon cancer secondary to dysplasia and possible genetic mutations linked to mucosal injury and repair. A history of previous adenomatous polyps as well as colon cancer is also risk factors. Breast cancer or a history of breast cancer is a risk factor for colon cancer secondary to shared environmental or hormonal factors. Previous radiation of the pelvis may cause mutations that increase risk. Diabetes may be a risk factor because insulin appears to modulate cellular proliferation in the colon. Acromegaly is a possible risk factor because growth hormone has been linked to proliferation of adenomas and cancers.

Clinical Presentation

Unfortunately, symptoms are more common and predominate late in the course of colon cancer and include abdominal pain, rectal bleeding, a change in bowel habits, and weight loss. A change in bowel habits may be either diarrhea or constipation; however, change in bowel habits typically represents colon cancer as opposed to simply being due to chronically abnormal bowel habits. Colon cancer symptoms will be determined by the location of the tumor, the size of the tumor, and the extent of metastatic disease. Left-sided cancers tend to cause partial/complete obstruction as opposed to right-sided colon cancers.

Distal locations of colon cancer may exhibit rectal bleeding, as opposed to proximal cancers, in which the blood is mixed with stool and is occult. One sign of proximal colon cancer and bleeding may be the presence of iron-deficiency anemia without overt signs of rectal bleeding. Advanced metastatic colon cancer may present with cancer cachexia—weight loss, anorexia, muscle weakness, and malaise. Anemia may present with pallor, nail changes (koilonychias), glossitis, and cheilitis. Ascites, anasarca, or peripheral edema may indicate hypoalbuminemia. The presence of a Virchow node as well as hepatomegaly may indicate advanced disease.

Laboratory Abnormalities

A CBC is always indicated in colon cancer, because 50% of patients with cancer of the colon are anemic. Any iron-deficiency anemia of an undetermined cause requires a work-up for colon cancer. LFTs are usually normal in patients with colon cancer, although high-alkaline phosphatase or lactate dehydrogenase may be indicative of liver metastasis. The serum carcinoembryonic antigen level (CEA) is not considered a useful screening tool for cancer of the colon because of only moderate sensitivity. CEA level is typically quite high in advanced disease.

Unusual Clinical Syndromes

Cancer of the colon may result in obstruction of the colon, typically secondary to an exophytic tumor that is located inside the lumen or, less likely, from a volvulus or intussusception. The most common location for obstruction due to colon cancer is the sigmoid colon. The sigmoid has a narrow lumen and typically has hard stool. On rare occasions, cancer of the colon may perforate and thus result in acute peritonitis, or may wall off into an inflammatory mass or abscess. It is rare for cancer of the colon to result in ischemic colitis.

Histology

Colon cancer has an origin in mucosal polyps in the colon, with the two most typical forms being hyperplastic and adenomatous polyps. Hyperplastic polyps "contain an increased number of glandular cells with decreased cytoplasmic mucus, but lack nuclear hyperchromatism, stratification, or atypia." Adenomas are either tuberous or villous in nature. Studies have shown that almost all cancers of the colon originate from adenomas. Hyperplastic polyps have a slightly increased risk of developing into cancer of the colon; risk factors are large size, location in the right colon, adenoma within the polyp, and family history.

Recent Advances in the Molecular Genetics

Cancer of the colon is considered one of most understood cancers in terms of molecular genetics. Detailed studies of familial adenomatous polyposis (FAP) and hereditary nonpolyposis colon cancer (HNPCC) were the basis of breakthroughs in understanding molecular aspects of the more common (non-syndrome) form of cancer of the colon. Patients with FAP will develop numerous adenomas that eventually become colon cancer. This is inherited in an autosomal-dominant manner with a mutation of the APC gene on chromosome 5q. HNPCC is due to mutations of mismatch repair genes, with hMLH1 and hMSH2 being the most common.

Current Theory on the Molecular Biology

Currently, cancer of the colon is thought to be a result of genetic mutations that produce increasingly disordered DNA replication and increased colonic cell replication. The result of increasingly disordered DNA replication secondary to increased genetic mutations is the following transition: normal mucosa to benign adenoma to high-grade dysplasia to frank carcinoma. 15% of sporadic cancers of the colon are secondary to mutations of the mismatch repair genes. 80% of sporadic cancers of the colon are secondary to APC mutation. APC gene mutations are also thought to be the cause of 50% of sporadic adenomas.

Pathology

The microscopic appearance of colon cancer is characterized as either well differentiated, moderately well-differentiated, or poorly differentiated, depending upon the degree of normal glandular and cytological structures that are present. 20% of colon cancers are considered to be poorly differentiated and have a poor prognosis. 15% of colon cancers are considered to be mucinous, or colloid, and are very aggressive tumors. 65% of cancers of the colon are found distal to the splenic flexure with 35% being located proximal to the sigmoid colon. Colon cancer may be found in a pedunculated polyp, sessile polyp, mass, or stricture.

Stages

Carcinoma-in-situ (high-grade dysplasia) is localized to the mucosa but does not go through the muscularis mucosa. Invasive colon cancer is typically classified into stages A through D (Dukes classification). Stage A shows penetration into the submucosa. Stage B1 exhibits penetration into the muscularis propria, and Stage B2 has penetration into the serosa. Stage C exhibits metastases to regional lymph nodes. Stage D is characterized by distant metastases. Colon cancer is also staged by the TMN classification (tumor-node-metastases) wherein T=depth of the primary tumor, N=presence of local lymph node metastases, and M=presence of distant metastases.

Screening and Diagnostic Tests

Fecal occult blood testing is only moderately sensitive and of low specificity in detecting colon cancer. However, an unexplained positive fecal occult blood test in patients over 40 requires further diagnostic work-up. Barium enema is moderately sensitive in detecting colon cancer as well. This test is considered even less sensitive in the detection of colonic polyps. Sigmoidoscopy does not enable visualization of the proximal half of the colon and thus is thought to be rather insensitive. Colonoscopy is the suggested test for screening of those over age 50 with an average risk of colon cancer.

Colonoscopy

"Colonoscopy is highly sensitive at detecting large (greater than 1 cm) colonic polyps, with a miss rate of only 6%, and is moderately sensitive at detecting diminutive (less than 0.6 cm) polyps with a miss rate of about 27%." Polyps are usually missed near the hepatic and sigmoid flexures (due to the sharp turns at these sites), at areas with significant spasm (typically in the sigmoid or in areas of significant diverticulosis), and areas with a large amount of stool secondary to a poor prep. Colon cancers are not often missed because they are usually larger than adenomatous polyps. The following are acute indications for colonoscopy to exclude adenomas, colon cancer, or other disease of the colon: fecal occult blood, iron-deficiency anemia, hematochezia, melena (with non-diagnostic EGD), *Streptococcus bovis* bacteremia, sigmoidoscopy findings of polyps in the colon, adenocarcinoma metastatic to the liver with an unknown primary, change in bowel habits in the elderly, follow-up after colonoscopic removal of a large sessile proximal colonic polyp, abnormal radiologic study (barium enema, virtual colonoscopy) suggestive of colon cancer, colonic stricture, dye injection to label a malignant polyp for subsequent surgical removal, and intraoperative colonoscopy to localize a lesion for surgical removal.

Other Testing

CT of the abdomen is the typical modality utilized to obtain information about the abdomen in patients with colon cancer and is rather accurate in demonstrating hepatic metastases. CT of the abdomen is much more sensitive for large liver lesions than smaller liver lesions. CT scanning of the abdomen is considered to be only moderately accurate in T staging. MRI of the abdomen is much more sensitive, especially for the detection of smaller liver metastases, than the CT scan. MRI is also thought to be more specific for liver lesions than CT scan.

Rectal Cancer

98% of cancers of the rectum are adenocarcinomas, 0.4% are carcinoid, 1.3% are lymphomas, and 0.3% are sarcomas. There have been very rare cases of squamous cell carcinoma of the rectum. The American Cancer Society estimated in 2009 that colorectal cancer caused 9% of all cancer deaths. Mortality rates at 1 year and 5 years are 83% and 64%, respectively. When detected early, the 5-year survival rate is approximately 90%. Over 90% of colorectal cancer occurs in patients over the age of 50.

Often, rectal cancer is asymptomatic and is discovered incidentally upon digital or proctoscope examination. 60% of patients with cancer of the rectum present with rectal bleeding. Such bleeding may also be associated with the passage of mucus. 43% of patients experience a change in bowel habits, which is often noted as the onset of diarrhea. Cancer that is located in the lower aspect of the rectum will cause symptoms of tenesmus and incomplete emptying. 26% have a positive fecal occult blood test while 20% have abdominal pain.

Decision-Making Process for Surgical Treatment

It is important to think about the following when determining an appropriate treatment plan for rectal cancer: surgical intent, functional outcome, and the preservation of anal continence and GU functions. It is important to attempt to achieve a cure, because the risk of recurrence is high in rectal cancer. The current standard of care is sphincter-saving procedures. There are multiple factors that influence sphincter preservation, such as the training of the surgeon, the volume of cases of the surgeon, and the use of neo-adjuvant chemotherapy. It is crucial to consider factors that may be associated with difficult sphincter preservation.

Factors Involved in Considering the Type of Surgical Procedure

The following factors generally indicate a difficult sphincter preservation: male gender, morbid obesity, incontinence demonstrated preoperatively, direct involvement of the muscles of the anal sphincter with tumor, and bulky cancers located within 5 cm of the anal verge. The following factors may indicate a successful local excision of rectal cancer: tumor located in the lower rectum, tumor that involves less than one-third of the circumference of the rectum, tumor that is mobile (exophytic/polypoid lesion), tumor less than 3 cm in size, T1 lesions, and low-grade tumor with negative nodes (both clinically and radiographically).

Irritable Bowel Syndrome

Irritable bowel syndrome is considered a functional GI disorder in that it is characterized by abdominal pain and altered bowel habits, with a lack of definite organic pathology. Irritable bowel syndrome was once thought to be a diagnosis of exclusion but is now a syndrome with a large differential diagnosis. Some of the traditional theories about irritable bowel syndrome include altered GI motility, visceral hyperalgesia, and psychopathology. At present, some patients have been found to have microscopic inflammation, which is considered to be a groundbreaking find, since irritable bowel syndrome has traditionally been thought to be a disorder without distinct pathology.

Etiologies

One of the proposed etiologies of irritable bowel syndrome is an abnormal transit in the GI tract and a heightened sense of normal GI motility. Approximately 33% of patients with irritable bowel syndrome may be noted to have an altered GI transit. Patients that have predominately constipation symptoms may be noted to have a delay in GI motility; patients that have predominately diarrhea symptoms may be noted to have a more rapid GI transit time than healthy controls. Enteric infection may contribute to hyperreactivity of the musculature of the colon, which may persist and contribute to irritable bowel syndrome.

Epidemiology

The prevalence of irritable bowel disease is thought to be 10-20% with an annual incidence of 1-2%. In the United States and in Europe, similar frequencies of irritable bowel syndrome are noted among ethnic and racial lines. In Asia and in Africa, lower prevalence of irritable bowel syndrome is noted. In Western societies, women are 2-3 times more likely than men to have irritable bowel syndrome. In the subcontinent of India, men comprise 70-80% of the cases of irritable bowel syndrome. 50% of patients with irritable bowel have onset of symptoms prior to age 35.

Clinical Presentation

A careful and precise history is essential in the diagnosis of irritable bowel syndrome. Altered bowel habits is a common symptom. The constipation noted in irritable bowel syndrome is described as small, hard, and narrow stools with painful or infrequent passage of stool, and the constipation will not respond to laxative administration. The diarrhea noted in irritable bowel syndrome is characterized by small amounts of loose stool that is preceded by urgency and increased frequency of defecation. Diffuse abdominal pain is a symptom and typically is located in the left lower quadrant.

Symptoms That Are Inconsistent

Symptoms that are not consistent with irritable bowel syndrome should alert the physician to search for possible organic etiologies. Such symptoms include the onset of irritable bowel symptoms in patients who are middle-aged or older, the acute onset of symptoms (irritable bowel syndrome is characterized by a chronicity of symptoms), symptoms that are progressive, symptoms that occur at night, anorexia or involuntary weight loss, fever, rectal bleeding, painless diarrhea, symptoms of steatorrhea, symptoms that are consistent with a lactose intolerance or a fructose intolerance, and gluten intolerance.

Rome III Criteria

The Rome III criteria for the diagnosis of irritable bowel syndrome "require that the patients have had recurrent abdominal pain or discomfort at least 3 days a month during the previous 3 months that is associated with 2 or more of the following: relieved by defecation, onset associated with a change in stool frequency, and onset associated with a change in stool form or appearance." "Supporting symptoms include the following: altered stool frequency, altered stool form, altered stool passage (straining and/or urgency), mucorrhea, abdominal bloating, and subjective distention." There are also 4 bowel patterns that may be noted in irritable bowel syndrome.

Differential Diagnosis

Physicians should think about the following disorders in the differential diagnosis of irritable bowel syndrome: fructose intolerance, gastrinoma, infectious colitis, adverse effects of drugs, secretory diarrhea, VIPoma, abdominal angina, anxiety disorders, bacterial overgrowth syndrome, biliary colic, biliary disease, celiac sprue, chronic mesenteric ischemia, collagenous and lymphocytic colitis, adenocarcinoma of the colon, endometriosis, allergies to foods, bacterial gastroenteritis, viral gastroenteritis, giardiasis, hypercalcemia, hyperthyroidism, hypothyroidism, inflammatory bowel disease, cancer of the small intestine, mesenteric artery/venous thrombosis, pancreatic cancer, chronic pancreatitis, pheochromocytoma, acute intermittent porphyria, lead toxicity, and ulcerative colitis.

Work-Up

In 2009, the American College of Gastroenterologists (ACG) established a position statement on the diagnosis and management of irritable bowel syndrome. ACG noted that laboratory or radiologic testing is not recommended in patients under age 50 unless "alarm symptoms" are present. Alarm symptoms are weight loss, the presence of iron-deficiency anemia, and a family history of inflammatory bowel disease, celiac sprue, or colorectal cancer. A CBC is typically needed to look for anemia, inflammation, or infection. Metabolic panels are also needed to look for metabolic disorders and/or electrolyte disorders—especially in patients with diarrhea.

Functional Bloating

Functional bloating is defined as "a recurrent sensation of Abdominal distension that may or may not be associated with measurable distention, but is not part of another functional bowel or gastroduodenal disorder." The diagnostic criteria for functional bloating must be met for the previous 3 months, with the onset of symptoms at least 6 months before diagnosis, and must include both of the following: "recurrent feeling of bloating or visible distention at least 3 days per month for 3 months, and insufficient criteria for a diagnosis of functional dyspepsia, IBS, or other functional GI disorder."

Functional Constipation

Functional constipation is defined "as a functional bowel disorder that presents as persistently difficult, infrequent, or seemingly incomplete defecation, which does not meet IBS criteria." The diagnostic criteria for functional constipation must include 2 or more of the following: "straining during at least 25% of defecations, lumpy or hard stools in at least 25% of defecations, sensation of incomplete evacuation for at least 25% of defecations, sensation of anorectal obstruction/blockage for at least 25% of defecations, manual maneuvers to facilitate at least 25% of defecations (e.g., digital evacuation, support of the pelvic floor), fewer than 3 defecations per week, loose stools are rarely present without the use of laxatives, and insufficient criteria for IBS."

Functional Diarrhea

Functional diarrhea is defined as "a continuous or recurrent syndrome characterized by the passage of loose (mushy) or watery stools without abdominal pain or discomfort." The diagnostic criterion for functional diarrhea must be fulfilled for the last 3 months with the onset of symptoms at least 6 months prior to diagnosis. The diagnostic criterion for functional diarrhea is "loose (mushy) or watery stools without pain occurring in at least 75% of stools." It is very important to obtain a complete dietary history since provocative foods (for example, foods that contain sorbitol) can be avoided as a measure to decrease symptoms.

Liver

Hepatic Disorders in HIV Infection

Most patients with HIV infection will exhibit hepatobiliary symptoms during the course of the disease, with 50% having hepatomegaly and/or jaundice, and with 80% having abnormal LFTs. Hepatic disease is only rarely a cause of death in advanced HIV infection; most hepatic disorders are a result of opportunistic infection or neoplasm. MAC is the most typical opportunistic organism seen on liver biopsy that causes hepatic disease in HIV infection and should be carefully distinguished from lesions caused by tuberculosis (TB). Extra-pulmonary TB may occur in more than 50% of infected patients.

Peliosis hepatitis is a bacterial infection caused by *Bartonella henselae* that results in elevated transaminases, skin lesions, fever, sweats, shaking rigors, RUQ pain, and bony pain from lytic lesions. It is treated with a prolonged course of erythromycin, doxycycline, ciprofloxacin, or anti-tuberculosis medications. Fungal infections of the liver often only occur with disseminated disease and usually present with nonspecific findings such as hepatic enlargement, fever, and high alkaline phosphatase levels. Pneumocystis is the most typical protozoal infection pathogen seen in HIV infection and involves hepatic involvement in 38% of patients.

HBV and HIV Infection

90% of homosexual patients with HIV infection demonstrate seropositivity for past or present infection with HBV, with similar rates seen in IV drug abusers with both infections. Immunocompetent patients with acute HBV infection have a 95% rate of HBV clearance; whereas 50% of HIV-infected patients will go on to develop chronic HBV infection. A large number of patients with co-infection of HIV and HBV are chronic carriers and have highly infectious body fluids.

HCV and HIV Infection

Both HIV and HCV have a parenteral mode of transmission and typically may be seen in IV drug abusers. Immunocompetent patients infected with HCV usually have a prolonged course of the disease, and liver failure results in only a small percentage of these patients. The course of HCV disease is accelerated in patients with HIV infection. The risk of hepatic disease is greatly elevated in patients with HIV infection. HIV infection, as with HBV disease, ultimately determines the morbidity and mortality in this patient population, however. Alpha-interferon is the only medication presently approved by the FDA for treatment.

Biliary Disease Seen in HIV Infection

There are three categories of biliary tract disorders seen in HIV infection: non-HIV disorders of the bile duct, acalculous cholecystitis, and AIDS cholangiopathy. Non-HIV disorders of the bile duct include cholelithiasis, stricture, or periampullary cancers of the bile duct. Acalculous cholecystitis is rare but has been associated with infection with CMV or *Cryptosporidium*; most patients are young and present with RUQ pain and abnormal LFTs. Previous infection with CMV or *C. parvum* is frequently present, as well as sclerosing cholangitis and papillary stenosis of the distal common bile duct. Cholecystectomy is often beneficial.

Acute Liver Failure

Acute liver failure may be fulminant hepatic failure or may be sub-fulminant hepatic failure. Acute hepatic failure is very rare and results in rapid decline of hepatic function, which leads to coagulopathy and significant mental status changes. The term *acute hepatic failure* is utilized to delineate the development of coagulopathy and any degree of encephalopathy in a patient that does not have pre-existing cirrhosis with a length of illness less than 26 weeks. Fulminant hepatic failure typically describes encephalopathy within 8 weeks of symptom onset in a previously healthy patient.

Acute Hepatic Failure

The primary cause of morbidity and mortality in patients with acute hepatic failure is the development of cerebral edema. Etiologic factors for cerebral edema are not clearly understood but may include elevated ammonia levels. Cerebral edema may also be secondary to both cytotoxic and vasogenic aspects. Cytotoxic edema is secondary to impairment of cerebral cellular osmoregulation, which results in astrocyte edema (glutamine accumulation is the primary cause). Vasogenic edema is a result of increased brain blood flow and increased brain blood volume and causes a disruption in cerebral autoregulation, possibly mediated via high systemic levels of nitric oxide.

Causes

The most common causes of acute hepatic failure are acetaminophen hepatotoxicity and idiosyncratic drug reactions. 15% of acute hepatic failure cases have no definitive causal mechanism. Hepatitis A and B cause most cases of acute hepatic failure secondary to viral hepatitis. Hepatitis C is a rare cause of acute liver failure; however, hepatitis D (co-infection or superinfection with hepatitis B) may result in fulminant hepatic failure. Endemic cases of hepatitis E, especially in pregnant women, may result in fulminant hepatic failure. Unusual causes include CMV, hemorrhagic fever viruses, herpes simplex, paramyxovirus, and EBV.

Pregnancy

0.008% of pregnancies result in acute fatty liver of pregnancy, which typically occurs in the third trimester. Preeclampsia occurs in 50% of pregnancies. Acute fatty liver of pregnancy often causes fulminant hepatic failure. Pregnant patients who contract hepatitis E commonly develop fulminant hepatic failure, which is typically fatal. Hepatitis E should be considered in patients who travel to or live in the Middle East, India, and Mexico. It is rare in the United States. HELLP syndrome is characterized by hemolysis, elevated liver enzymes, and low platelets. HELLP syndrome occurs in 0.1 to 0.6% of pregnancies, is associated with preeclampsia, and can occasionally cause hepatic failure.

Drug-Related Hepatotoxicity

A large number of drugs, both prescription and illicit, can cause acute hepatic failure. In the United States, unintentional acetaminophen overdose is the cause of 48% of cases of hepatic failure, with 44% of cases being secondary to intentional overdose. Chronic alcohol use has been shown to increase hepatotoxicity from acetaminophen as a result of depleted glutathione stores. The following medications have been linked to idiosyncratic hypersensitivity reactions and hepatic failure: antibiotics (ampicillin-clavulanate, ciprofloxacin, doxycycline, erythromycin, INH, nitrofurantoin, and tetracycline), amitriptyline, nortriptyline, phenytoin, valproate, halothane, certain statins, and NSAIDs.

Drugs and Toxins and Vascular Disorders

Ecstasy and cocaine have been known to cause hepatic failure. Herbal medications that can cause hepatic failure include ginseng, pennyroyal oil, Teucrium polium, chaparral or germander tea, and kava-kava. Dose-related toxicity of the following toxins may cause hepatic failure: *Amanita phalloides* mushroom toxin, *Bacillus cereus* toxin, cyanobacteria toxin, organic solvents such as carbon tetrachloride, and yellow phosphorus. Vascular causes of hepatic failure include ischemic hepatitis, hepatic vein thrombosis (Budd-Chiari syndrome), veno-occlusive disease of the liver, portal vein thrombosis, and thrombosis of the hepatic artery—especially posttransplant.

Other Causes

Other causes of hepatic failure may be metabolic causes, such as alpha-1-antitrypsin deficiency, fructose intolerance, galactosemia, lecithin-cholesterol acyltransferase deficiency, Reye's syndrome, tyrosinemia, and Wilson disease. There are various malignancies that may cause acute hepatic failure. Malignancies that my result in acute hepatic failure include hepatocellular carcinoma or cholangiocarcinoma (primary liver tumors); extensive liver metastases; or infiltration from adenocarcinoma from such primaries as breast, lung, and melanoma (most common), or from lymphoma or leukemia. Other causes of acute hepatic failure are adult-onset: Still disease, heat stroke, and primary graft malfunction in liver transplants.

Prognosis

Prior to advances in orthotopic liver transplantation, mortality for acute hepatic failure exceeded 80%. In the United States, 6% of liver transplants are performed for acute or fulminant hepatic failure. The primary determining prognostic factors in acute hepatic failure are cause and complications. For example, acute hepatic failure secondary to acetaminophen overdose has a better prognosis than cases of acute hepatic failure from undetermined causes, while the presence of grade 3 or 4 encephalopathy is a poor prognostic indicator. Mortality risk is higher with complications such as cerebral edema, renal failure, ARDS, infection, and coagulopathy.

Clinical Presentation

The history is always the most important element in a patient encounter, but it is vital to address the following aspects with a patient in acute hepatic failure: timing—when jaundice and encephalopathy began; use of alcohol; all medication use—prescription, herbal, or illicit; any family history of hepatic disease—especially Wilson disease; viral hepatitis risk factors—travel, blood transfusions, sexual contacts, occupation, and body piercings/tattoos; hepatic toxin exposure—mushrooms; organic solvents; fireworks (containing phosphorus); and the presence of any complications such as renal failure, seizures, coagulopathy, or infection. On physical examination, one must carefully assess mental status and any signs of chronic hepatic disease.

Clinical Grading

Grading of hepatic encephalopathy is based upon the following parameters: level of consciousness, personality and intellect, neurologic signs, and EEG abnormalities. Grade 0 hepatic encephalopathy is characterized by normal level of consciousness, personality, and intellect, with no neurologic or EEG abnormalities; sub-clinical encephalopathy exhibits abnormalities only upon psychometric testing. Grade 1 hepatic encephalopathy is characterized by sleep reversal and restlessness, agitation, forgetfulness, irritability, mild confusion, tremor, apraxia, poor coordination, altered handwriting, and 5-Hz triphasic waves on EEG. Grade 2 hepatic encephalopathy is characterized by lethargy with slow responses, disorientation, inhibition loss or inappropriate behavior, asterixis, ataxia, and triphasic waves on EEG. Grade 3 hepatic encephalopathy is characterized by sleepiness and confusion, asterixis, Babinski, hyperactive reflexes, and triphasic waves on EEG. Grade 4 hepatic encephalopathy is characterized by coma, decerebration, and delta activity on EEG.

Complications

Seizures may be secondary to the underlying cause of hepatic failure or may be a result of intracranial hemorrhage or increased intracranial hypertension and are typically treated with phenytoin, since sedatives make it more difficult to accurately assess mental status changes. Altered coagulation status may result in hemorrhage and often presents with GI bleeding from varices that are due to portal hypertension. Coagulopathy and hemorrhage are treated by FFP or transfusions. Infections, either bacterial or fungal, require the use of surveillance cultures, and empiric broad-spectrum coverage may be indicated. Acute renal failure may be secondary to dehydration, hepatorenal syndrome, or acute tubular necrosis.

Diagnostic Considerations

The most important diagnostic aspect in acute hepatic failure is to attempt to identify the cause. The prognosis of acute hepatic failure is dependent upon the causal mechanism. CBC will often demonstrate thrombocytopenia; protime/INR is used to assess the presence and/or degree of coagulopathy. LFT will typically show extensive elevations of AST, ALT, SGOT, and SGPT secondary to extensive hepatocellular necrosis. Serum bilirubin levels will be high and will climb as the acute hepatic failure gets worse. Serum ammonia will be greatly increased; arterial ammonia level is considered to be the most accurate.

Treatment and Management

The treatment and management of acute hepatic failure entails intensive supportive care. Most patients will have circulatory dysfunction; thus, it is paramount to carefully monitor fluid balance and hemodynamic parameters. Monitoring for infection and electrolyte imbalance is also crucial, as is surveillance for bleeding and maintenance of proper nutritional support. Patients with acute hepatic failure who progress to grade 3 encephalopathy will require NG tube placement and airway protection. An infusion of propofol may be advantageous for intubation, to decrease the cerebral blood flow, and to prevent intracranial hypertension.

Liver Transplantation

Liver transplantation is the definitive treatment for acute hepatic failure. As a general rule, the following list of complications of hepatic failure are indicative of a need for transplant: "recurrent variceal hemorrhage, intractable ascites, spontaneous bacterial peritonitis, refractory encephalopathy, severe jaundice, exacerbated synthetic dysfunction, sudden deterioration, and fulminant hepatic failure." Contraindications for liver transplantation include active spontaneous bacterial peritonitis, other active infection, severe and advanced cardiac or pulmonary disease, extrahepatic malignancy that does not meet criteria for cure, current abuse of alcohol or substance abuse, and the inability to follow protocols for immunosuppression.

Encephalopathy and Cerebral Edema

Patients with acute hepatic failure and encephalopathy or cerebral edema need the head of the bed elevated to 30 degrees with minimal stimulation. Valsalva-like maneuvers must be avoided in order to prevent increases in intracranial pressure. Administration of lactulose may aid in decreasing ammonia levels; care is needed to prevent aspiration, however. An intracranial pressure monitor (ICP) is often placed in patients with grade 3 or 4 encephalopathy to facilitate the recognition of cerebral edema. The typical signs of elevated intracranial pressure—hypertension, bradycardia, and irregular breathing—are not always present.

Intracranial Hypertension

The initial management of intracranial hypertension is osmotic diuresis with mannitol administration. Mannitol administration is a short-term tool and can lead to fluid overload in patients with renal failure, thus necessitating dialysis. Hyperventilation to blow off carbon dioxide may also be used as a short-term measure, since low carbon dioxide will rapidly lower ICP as a result of cerebral vasoconstriction that causes a decrease in cerebral blood flow. Refractory intracranial hypertension is occasionally treated with the use of hypertonic saline, barbiturates, and hypothermia. Possible risks of hypothermia include elevated infection risk, coagulopathy, and cardiac arrhythmia.

Treatment and Management of Acetaminophen Toxicity

Acetaminophen toxicity or overdose is treated with N-acetylcysteine (NAC). The protective mechanisms of N-acetylcysteine are as follows: NAC will stop the formation and accumulation of N-acetyl-p-benzoquinone imine (NAPQI). NAPQI is a free radical that will bind with intracellular proteins and cause toxicity. NAC also elevates glutathione stores and competes with NAPQI as a glutathione substitute, and will facilitate sulfate conjugation. NAC also works as an anti-inflammatory and antioxidant agent with positive inotropic and vasodilation effects. Such effects of NAC will enhance microcirculation and improve tissue oxygen delivery.

Viral Hepatitis

The term *hepatitis* is used to describe inflammation of the liver and may be secondary to alcohol, medications, autoimmune disorders, metabolic disorders, and viruses. 50% of the cases of hepatitis in the United States are secondary to viral hepatitis. Etiologic agents of viral hepatitis include hepatitis A virus, hepatitis B virus, hepatitis C virus, hepatitis D virus, and hepatitis E virus. Other causes of viral hepatitis are CMV, adenovirus, Epstein-Barr virus, and herpes simplex virus. 95% of the cases of acute viral hepatitis in the United States are due to HAV, HBV, HCV, HDV (requires coexisting HBV infection), and HEV.

Viral Transmission Patterns

Fecal-oral transmission is typically seen with HAV and HEV. Parenteral transmission is commonly seen with HBV, HCV, HDV, HGV, and sometimes with HAV. Sexual transmission is noted with HBV, HCV, and HDV. Perinatal transmission is noted with HBV, HCV, and HDV. Sporadic transmission may occasionally be seen with HBV and with HCV. Hepatitis A virus is the most typical cause of acute viral hepatitis in the United States. Hepatitis C virus is the most typical cause of chronic viral hepatitis in the United States. Currently, it is unknown if hepatitis G virus is pathogenic.

Natural History of Acute Viral Hepatitis

Acute viral hepatitis may have a subclinical presentation, may be self-limited and symptomatic, or may progress to fulminant liver failure. Acute viral hepatitis secondary to hepatitis A or hepatitis B is typically symptomatic, while acute viral hepatitis due to hepatitis C may be either asymptomatic or symptomatic. The common symptoms of acute viral hepatitis are fatigue, anorexia, nausea, and vomiting. Fulminant hepatic failure may occur in 1% of cases of acute viral hepatitis secondary to hepatitis A or hepatitis B. A typical cause of fulminant hepatic failure due to acute viral hepatitis in Asia is hepatitis E.

Natural History of Chronic Viral Hepatitis

An evolution to chronic viral hepatitis is noted in 90-95% of neonates with acute hepatitis B infection, in 5% of adults with acute hepatitis B infection, and in up to 85% of cases of acute hepatitis C infection. In 20% of those with chronic hepatitis B or chronic hepatitis C, cirrhosis will develop. Some patients with chronic viral hepatitis will be asymptomatic for life while other patients with chronic viral hepatitis note symptoms of mild to severe fatigue and dyspepsia. The clinical spectrum of chronic hepatitis evolving into cirrhosis may take years.

Hepatitis A

Hepatitis A virus is a picornavirus and is usually transmitted via a fecal-oral means. There have been very rare cases of transmission of hepatitis A via transfusion or inoculation. Hepatitis A is relatively common in Africa, Asia, and Central and South America; the Middle East has a high prevalence as well. Improved sanitation in the United States and in developed nations has lowered the overall prevalence of hepatitis A to less than 50% of the population. The incubation period for hepatitis A is from 15-45 days; the virus is excreted fecally prior to the onset of symptoms.

Symptoms

Common symptoms include several weeks of malaise, anorexia, nausea, and vomiting, and high levels of aminotransferases. Jaundice may be a finding in more severe cases of hepatitis A infection. High levels of aminotransferases is a classic finding, but some patients demonstrate cholestatic hepatitis, which is characterized by high levels of alkaline phosphatase. Fewer than 1% of hepatitis A infections end

in fulminant hepatic failure. Infection with hepatitis A is not considered to be persistent and does not ever result in the development of chronic viral hepatitis. Acute hepatitis A infection is demonstrated by the presence of IgM anti-HAV.

Prevention

The first vaccine for hepatitis A was approved by the FDA in 1995. The hepatitis A vaccine is recommended for anyone traveling to endemic areas, homosexual men, illicit drug abusers, and children living in endemic states with a high rate of hepatitis A infection. As of 2006, the FDA is recommending that all children receive vaccination at age 1 year. Other populations that should receive the vaccine for hepatitis A include those with occupational exposure, patients that need clotting factor treatments, patients with chronic hepatic disease, and patients who are awaiting or have received liver transplants.

Hepatitis B Infection

5% of the population of the world is chronically infected with hepatitis B; 20% will progress to hepatocellular carcinoma. Hepatitis B infection is the 10th leading cause of death in the world. Most of the cases of hepatitis B worldwide are secondary to perinatal transmission. Hepatitis B virus is much more easily transmitted via sexual activity than HIV or hepatitis C virus; 50% of the cases of hepatitis B infection in the United States are secondary to sexual transmission. 20% of the cases in the United States are secondary to IV drug use.

Natural History

Hepatitis B has an incubation period ranging from 40-150 days; the infection may be mild or can progress to fulminant hepatic failure. Following an acute hepatitis B infection, 90-95% of adults and 5-10% of neonates will develop antibodies are go on to completely recover. 5% of adults and 90-95% of neonates develop chronic hepatitis B. An inactive carrier state occurs with the seroconversion from HBeAg positive status to HBeAg negative status; inactive carriers are thought to be infectious through parenteral or through sexual contact. 10-30% of carriers develop chronic hepatitis.

Hepatocellular Carcinoma

Approximately 1 million cases of hepatocellular carcinoma occur annually in the world with the majority secondary to hepatitis B infection. Cirrhosis, as opposed to other hepatic disease, is not a prerequisite for developing hepatocellular carcinoma. The causal mechanism for the development of hepatocellular carcinoma in patients with hepatitis B infection is thought to be integration of the virus into the genome, with subsequent oncogene activation or inhibition of tumor suppression genes.

Hepatitis C Infection

The hepatitis C virus is a flavivirus that has one serotype and numerous genotypes. Genotype 1b is the most typical genotype seen in the United States. The genotypic variability is one of the main reasons for the difficulty in creating an effective vaccine against hepatitis C. Hepatitis C has a prevalence of 0.5-2% in the world; in the United States, 4% of acute cases of hepatitis C are secondary to transfusion of blood products. It is estimated that 60% of new cases of hepatitis C are due to drug use with sharing of drug paraphernalia.

Natural History

The incubation period for hepatitis C is 8 weeks; most of the cases of acute hepatitis C are asymptomatic. Symptomatic cases of acute hepatitis C tend to be mild in nature. About 75-80% of patients with new hepatitis C infections stay viremic and may progress to chronic hepatic disease. 20% of patients with chronic hepatitis C infection develop cirrhosis, but this process may require 10-40 years to be demonstrated. Patients with chronic hepatitis C infection and cirrhosis have a greater risk of hepatocellular carcinoma, especially if co-infection with hepatitis B is present as well.

Pyogenic Hepatic Abscess

Hepatic abscesses may be pyogenic, fungal, amebic, or echinococcal in origin. Most hepatic abscesses are pyogenic (80%) and are typically secondary to cholangitis. Common pathogens that cause pyogenic liver abscess are *E. coli, Klebsiella, Pseudomonas, Proteus, Staph aureus, Enterococcus, Strep viridans, Bacteroides,* and *Fusobacterium*. Uncommon pathogens include *Enterobacter, Citrobacter, Serratia*, beta-hemolytic strep, anaerobic strep, *Clostridium*, and *Lactobacilli*. The treatment for pyogenic abscess is drainage and antibiotics; most are able to be drained in a percutaneous manner. If untreated, pyogenic abscess is almost always fatal—mortality rates are 10-20% with treatment.

Amebic Hepatic Abscess

The most typical extra-intestinal manifestation of *E. histolytica* is an amebic hepatic abscess. Amebic hepatic abscess is more common in men with a 10:1 predominance. The common mechanism to acquire amebiasis is to ingest the cysts via a fecal-oral route of transmission. Most infections are due to contaminated water/vegetable, food contaminated by fertilizer/carrier hands, or by direct transmission. The most typical signs of amebic abscess are fever, RUQ pain, and hepatomegaly. Most patients are simply treated with amebicidal medications, though some will need aspiration, percutaneous drainage, or open surgical drainage. Mortality rates are 0-18% and risk of rupture is 3-17%.

Fungal Hepatic Abscess

Approximately 10% of hepatic abscesses are fungal in origin. 80% of hepatic fungal abscesses are secondary to *Candida albicans* and other forms of *Candida*. Fungal abscesses of the liver are typically multiple and are usually demonstrated in patients who are immunocompromised. The treatment of fungal hepatic abscess is systemic antifungal therapy and drainage by either simple aspiration, percutaneous method, or open surgical method. Amphotericin B is the typical antifungal agent that is used secondary to the broad spectrum of activity but voriconazole or caspofungin may also be used if the infection does not respond to amphotericin B or is aggressive.

Echinococcal Hepatic Abscess

Echinococcal hepatic abscess is due to a flat tapeworm that is transmitted to humans via contaminated vegetables or via contact with infected soil/animals. Medical treatment results in

30% cure rate. Medical treatment, therefore, is typically used in conjunction with surgical drainage. Medications to treat such an abscess are mebendazole and albendazole. Currently, praziquantel is being combined with albendazole as well. Uncomplicated echinococcal hepatic abscess has a morbidity rate of 20% and a mortality rate of 1%. Combined surgical and medical treatment is very successful, with recurrence rates of less than 10%.

Simple and Complex Hepatic Cysts

Most simple cysts are solitary and are not symptomatic. Simple cysts are usually less than 5 cm in size but can be as large as 20 cm. Symptoms from simple cysts are typically secondary to a mass effect, which usually is RUQ pain or early satiety but can be secondary to hemorrhage within the cyst itself or infection. Cysts greater than 5 cm that cause symptoms will need laparoscopic drainage or open cyst unroofing. Multiple cysts may be due to polycystic liver disease, which is autosomal dominant and associated with cysts in the kidney as well.

Hepatic Hemangioma

Hepatic hemangioma is typically discovered between the ages of 30 and 70 with a female-to-male ratio of 6:1. Hemangiomas originate from the endothelial lining of vessels and are linked to high estrogen, such as seen in puberty, pregnancy, oral contraceptive use, and treatment with androgens. Hepatic hemangiomas are typically not symptomatic and are less than 5 cm in size. Hepatic hemangiomas very rarely need surgical intervention because most do not cause symptoms, and the risk of rupture is minimal. If hepatic hemangiomas are symptomatic, simple surgical enucleation is commonly undertaken.

Focal Nodular Hyperplasia

The second most common benign solid tumor in the liver is focal nodular hyperplasia (8% of all hepatic tumors). Focal nodular hyperplasia usually occurs in women and presents in the 30-50 year age range. Most patients with focal nodular hyperplasia are asymptomatic but 10% have symptoms. The certainty of the diagnosis will determine if treatment is needed. If imaging studies are equivocal, a biopsy is needed. Nuclear medicine studies are often used to differentiate between focal nodular hyperplasia and hepatic adenoma because Kupffer cells are present in focal nodular hyperplasia and not in adenoma and have sulfa-colloid uptake.

Hepatic Adenoma

Hepatic adenoma is rare and is typically seen in women 20-40 years of age. Hepatic adenoma is strongly linked to the use of oral contraceptives and occurs in 3-4 out of 100,000 oral contraceptive users. 80% of hepatic adenomas are solitary and often demonstrate the presence of a pseudocapsule. Hepatic adenomas that are greater than 5 cm in size often cause symptoms and are hypervascular, which yields a moderately high chance of rupture. If a larger hepatic adenoma ruptures, one-third will be a rupture into the tumor with two-thirds rupturing into the peritoneum.

Primary Hepatic Cancer

Hepatocellular carcinoma usually results in death within 6-20 months and is often secondary to cirrhosis; however, 25% do not have evidence of cirrhosis. 2% of malignancies are due to hepatocellular carcinoma and the incidence is increasing, which is thought to be a result of hepatitis C, increasing obesity, and diabetes. It is the 5th most common cancer in men in the world and the 8th most common in women in the world. Surgical cure is possible but only in 5% of cases. Median length of survival is typically 6 months.

CLINICAL PRESENTATION

Most of the patients with hepatocellular carcinoma will have signs of advanced cirrhosis. Signs of advanced cirrhosis are itching, jaundice, splenic enlargement, bleeding from varices, cachexia, enlarged abdominal girth from occlusion of the portal vein by thrombosis with the rapid development of ascites, and occasional RUQ pain. On physical examination, patients with hepatocellular carcinoma will have hepatomegaly, jaundice, ascites, stigmata of alcoholism such as Dupuytren contracture and spider angiomata, asterixis, pedal edema, evidence of collateral veins in the peri-umbilical area, and enlargement of hemorrhoidal veins. Cirrhosis of any cause is a major risk factor in the development of hepatocellular carcinoma.

CAUSES

80% of patients who have pre-existing cirrhosis will develop hepatocellular carcinoma. Most cases of cirrhosis in the United States are secondary to alcohol, hepatitis C infection, and hepatitis B infection. 30% of cases of hepatocellular carcinoma in the United States are due to excessive alcohol use with the risk of this cancer being 1% annually in patients with decompensated cirrhosis. 20% of cases in the United States are secondary to chronic hepatitis B infection and 30% to hepatitis C infection.

Patients with hemochromatosis and concomitant cirrhosis have a greater risk of developing hepatocellular carcinoma, with 30% of deaths related to hemochromatosis being secondary to hepatocellular carcinoma. High dietary levels of aflatoxin (fungal contamination byproduct of food primarily found in sub-Saharan Africa, east and Southeast Asia) have a direct link to the development of hepatocellular carcinoma due to the DNA damage and the mutation caused to the p53 gene. Other rare causes of hepatocellular carcinoma are primary biliary cirrhosis, androgenic steroids, primary sclerosing cholangitis, 1-antitrypsin deficiency, Thorotrast radioactive contrast material, oral contraceptives, and porphyria cutanea tarda.

TMN STAGING CRITERIA AND THE CLIP SCORING SYSTEM

TMN staging for hepatocellular carcinoma: "T1—solitary tumor without vascular invasion, T2—solitary tumor with vascular invasion or multiple tumors none more than 5 cm, T3—multiple tumors more than 5 cm or tumor involving a major branch of the portal or hepatic vein, T4—tumor with direct invasion of adjacent organs other than the gallbladder or with perforation of visceral peritoneum. N0—no nodal involvement, N1—regional nodal involvement, M0—no distant metastases, M1—metastases presence beyond the liver."

CLIP scoring system: "score of 0-2 is assigned for each of the 4 features listed below: child-Pugh stage, tumor morphology, alpha-fetoprotein, and portal vein thrombosis."

TREATMENT

Prior to treatment for hepatocellular carcinoma, it is suggested to treat the complications of cirrhotic liver disease. Cirrhosis is treated with diuretics, paracentesis, lactulose, variceal banding, and antibiotics for SBP. A medical treatment regimen for hepatocellular carcinoma will be determined by the following: size of the tumors, number of the tumors, location of the tumors, presence of cirrhosis, comorbidity and surgical risk, status of the patency of the portal vein, and the presence of metastatic disease. The only chance for a cure is surgical resection or transplant, but only 5% of patients with hepatocellular carcinoma are transplant candidates.

ALCOHOLIC LIVER DISEASE

Alcoholic liver disease is also known as alcoholic hepatitis. Alcoholic liver disease is progressive and results in inflammatory injury to the liver and is secondary to longstanding heavy alcohol use.

Mild forms of alcoholic liver disease often do not present with symptoms; however, more severe forms may exhibit the following: fever, liver enlargement, leukocytosis, impairment of hepatic function such as coagulopathy/jaundice, and evidence of portal hypertension such as ascites and encephalopathy or variceal hemorrhage. If alcoholic liver disease is significant enough to result in acute hepatic encephalopathy, there is a great risk of death.

Metabolism of Ethanol

The primary location of ethanol metabolism is in the liver. There are 3 enzyme systems in the liver that serve to oxidize ethanol: the cytosolic alcohol dehydrogenase (ADH) system, microsomal-ethanol-oxidizing system (MEOS), and the peroxisomal catalase system. The agent for oxidation in the cytosolic alcohol dehydrogenase system is nicotinamide adenine dinucleotide or NAD. The oxidizing agent in the microsomal-ethanol-oxidizing system is nicotinamide adenine dinucleotide phosphate (NADPH) and molecular oxygen. The primary enzyme is this system is cytochrome P-450 2E1, which also functions to transform other drugs, such as acetaminophen; alcohol causes up-regulation of this enzyme. Hydrogen peroxide is the oxidizing agent in the peroxisomal catalase system. The final product of all three systems is acetaldehyde, which is the reactant that causes injury.

Epidemiology

The abuse of alcohol is the most typical cause of serious hepatic disease in Western societies with 1% of the population of the United States being affected. Alcoholism and alcoholic liver disease are more prevalent in certain minority populations. Death rates for alcoholic liver disease are far greater for non-whites than for whites; the non-white male death rate is 1.7 times greater than that for white men, 1.9 times greater than that for non-white women, and 4 times greater than that of white women. Women are much more susceptible to the effects of ethanol.

Prognosis

The primary determinants of the long-term prognosis for alcoholic liver disease are the presence of cirrhosis and continued alcohol use. Cessation of alcohol use results in improvement in liver function with resolution of the histologic aspects of acute alcoholic liver disease. Continuation of ethanol abuse will ultimately cause persistence of alcoholic liver disease with a progression to cirrhosis. In patients with severe alcoholic liver disease, the mortality rate is near 50%; in the absence of encephalopathy, jaundice, or coagulopathy, the mortality rate is less than 5%.

Clinical Presentation

It is, as always, crucial to obtain a detailed history regarding alcohol use. Some indications of heavy alcohol use may be a history of numerous motor vehicle accidents, DUI convictions, and poor interpersonal relationships. A genetic factor in alcoholism also has been noted, and it is important to ask about a history of alcoholism in a family member. Symptomatic alcoholic liver disease may present with nonspecific findings such as fever, nausea, or malaise. Some patients will present with impairment of hepatic function, signs of portal hypertension, hepatic encephalopathy (confusion/lethargy), or ascites.

Complications

Complications of alcoholic liver disease are essentially the same as those of cirrhosis. Variceal hemorrhage can be significant and requires resuscitation and immediate protection of the airway. Over 90% of variceal hemorrhage can be aborted with interventional endoscopy and the use of somatostatin or octreotide, which functions to decrease the portal system pressure. Hepatic encephalopathy portends a dire prognosis and is typically treated with supportive care, lactulose, or the use of non-absorbable antibiotics. Coagulopathy and thrombocytopenia are common in patients who present with variceal bleeding and are treated with fresh frozen plasma. Other issues may include ascites, spontaneous bacterial peritonitis, and iron overload.

Laboratory Findings

Findings on CBC may include neutrophilic leukocytosis, anemia (secondary to the direct marrow suppression of ethanol), increased mean corpuscular volume (MCV), thrombocytosis or thrombocytopenia. Liver function tests (LFT) show a characteristic pattern in alcoholic liver disease. Most hepatic diseases show relatively normal or only slightly increased AST with increased ALT; however, alcoholic liver disease exhibits moderately increased AST with normal or only slightly increased ALT. An AST/ALT ratio greater than 1 is almost always noted in alcoholic liver disease. Increased alkaline phosphatase is typically only mild. GGTP is extremely increased in alcoholic liver disease.

Histologic Findings

In the presence of alcoholic liver disease, the most striking location for injury is in the centrilobular (perivenular) areas—zone 3 of Rappaport. Hepatocytes appear balloon-like with necrosis. Typically, a focal accumulation of PMNs is also noted. lymphocytes can also be noted, typically in the portal tracts. Mallory bodies, which are ropy eosinophilic hyaline inclusions, are often noted in the perinuclear cytoplasm. Mallory bodies are thought to be a characteristic of alcoholic liver disease but have also been present in other disease states. Other findings may include macrovesicular steatosis, perivenular fibrosis, and cirrhosis.

Hepatic Vascular Disorders

The hepatic blood supply is dual in nature with the portal vein providing two-thirds of the supply and the hepatic artery providing the rest of the blood supply. The hepatic veins serve to drain the liver into the inferior vena cava. Although the liver has a dual blood supply and compensatory mechanisms (hepatic arterial buffer response), it may sustain injury from ischemia, impaired venous drainage, or specific vascular lesions. Ischemia may be secondary to decreased blood flow, decreased oxygen delivery, or increased metabolism. Impairment of venous drainage may be due to focal or diffuse obstruction. Specific vascular lesions can involve the hepatic artery, hepatic vein, or the portal vein.

Hepatic Ischemia

A diffuse ischemic process may result in ischemic hepatitis; a focal ischemic process may result in hepatic infarction or ischemic cholangiopathy; and hepatic infarction is secondary to issues with the hepatic artery. The most typical mechanisms for ischemic hepatitis are systemic in nature and include impairment of hepatic perfusion, hypoxemia, and an increased metabolic demand. Focal lesions of the hepatic blood supply are less likely causes. Such causes may include hepatic artery thrombosis as a result of liver transplant or portal thrombosis secondary to a sickle cell crisis. Treatment is typically focused upon the cause.

Congestive Hepatopathy

Congestive hepatopathy is also known as passive hepatic congestion and is secondary to diffuse venous congestion in the hepatic system that is commonly due to right-sided heart failure. Right-sided heart failure results in elevated central venous pressure. Elevated central venous pressure is then transmitted to the liver via the inferior vena cava and the hepatic veins. Chronic passive congestion will result in hepatocyte atrophy, sinusoid distention, and centrizonal fibrosis, which can turn into cardiac cirrhosis. Symptoms may include RUQ pain and hepatomegaly. Jaundice, ascites, and splenic enlargement may also be noted.

Disorders of the Hepatic Artery

Hepatic artery occlusion may be secondary to thrombosis from hypercoagulability, arteriosclerosis, vasculitis, emboli as a result of endocarditis, tumor, embolization procedures, iatrogenic secondary to surgical ligation, structural abnormalities such as hepatic artery aneurysm, eclampsia, cocaine use, and sickle cell crisis. The typical outcome of hepatic artery occlusion is hepatic infarct. An occlusion of the hepatic artery will result in symptoms if hepatic infarction or hepatic ischemia develops. Symptoms usually are RUQ pain, fever, nausea and vomiting, and jaundice. Diagnosis is typically via Doppler ultrasound that is followed by angiography. Treatment is based upon the cause.

Budd-Chiari Syndrome

Budd-Chiari syndrome is an obstruction of the venous outflow of extra-hepatic vessels with the most typical cause being a clot that obstructs the hepatic veins and the inferior vena cava. Etiology of the clots can be secondary to thrombotic disorders such as protein S/C deficiency, pregnancy, oral contraceptives, hematologic disorders such as polycythemia, inflammatory bowel disease, connective tissue disease, trauma, infection, or invasion of the hepatic vein secondary to tumor. Symptoms may be anywhere from asymptomatic to fulminant hepatic failure or cirrhosis. In the absence of treatment, most will die of hepatic failure in 3 years.

Sinusoidal Obstruction Syndrome

Sinusoidal obstruction syndrome is a form of veno-occlusive disease, which is typically the result of endothelial injury and results in non-thrombotic occlusion of the terminal hepatic venules and sinusoids. The resultant venous congestion will result in portal hypertension and cirrhosis. Typical etiologies include radiation, graft-versus-host disease, various medicinal teas and herbs, and toxins such as aflatoxin, azathioprine, and various chemotherapy agents. Diagnosis is typically via clinical examination, LFTs, ultrasound, and possible liver biopsy. Treatment is typically intensive supportive care and is directed at the underlying causal mechanism. For progressive disease, shunting or transplant may be undertaken.

Portal Vein Thrombosis

Typical causes of portal vein thrombosis may be grouped by age. Typical causes of portal vein thrombosis in infants are umbilical stump infection or omphalitis that is spread from the umbilical vein to the portal vein or congenital portal vein issues. Children may develop portal vein thrombosis as a result of acute appendicitis when infection is transmitted to the portal system. The causes of portal vein thrombosis in adults may be surgical such as post-splenectomy, hypercoagulopathy from protein S/C deficiency, pregnancy, myeloproliferative disorders, cancer, trauma, cirrhosis, and portal hypertension with resultant congestion and stasis.

Peliosis Hepatitis

Peliosis hepatitis is a condition in which numerous blood-filled cysts occur randomly in the liver and is usually not symptomatic. The blood-filled cysts associated with peliosis hepatitis often do not have cell linings and are amidst hepatocytes. The blood-filled cysts, however, may occasionally be lined with endothelial cells and are associated with dilated sinusoids, which may be a result of injury to the cells that line the hepatic sinusoids. Etiologies of peliosis hepatitis may be hormones such as anabolic steroids, oral contraceptives, glucocorticoids,

tamoxifen, vinyl chloride exposure, vitamin A, and azathioprine—especially in renal transplant recipients. Cysts may rarely rupture, which may cause hemorrhage or death.

Hepatorenal Syndrome

Hepatorenal syndrome is the onset of renal failure in patients with chronic hepatic disease. It may also develop in the setting of fulminant hepatitis, with ascites and portal hypertension. 40% of patients with cirrhosis and ascites will incur hepatorenal syndrome in the course of their hepatic disease. The renal failure associated with hepatorenal syndrome is not reversible unless liver transplant is performed. In hepatorenal syndrome, renal failure is the result of vasoconstriction in the renal circulation and concomitant systemic arteriolar vasodilation, with subsequent decreases in systemic vascular resistance and arterial hypotension.

Epidemiology

Hepatorenal syndrome happens in 10% of patients in the hospital for ascites and cirrhosis. In the case of decompensated cirrhosis, the chance of having hepatorenal syndrome is 8-20% per year and 40% at 5 years. There are 2 different types of hepatorenal syndrome. Type 1 demonstrates rapid progressive renal failure and is typically caused by spontaneous bacterial peritonitis. Type 1 occurs in 25% of patients who have spontaneous bacterial peritonitis. If untreated, most live only 2 weeks and almost all die after 10 weeks after renal failure occurs. Type 2 has a more stable course and usually occurs in those with relatively preserved hepatic function; survival is typically 3-6 months in these patients.

Hepatorenal Syndrome

Most of the causes of hepatorenal syndrome are related to the function of the circulatory system and the function of the renal system. Three critical risk factors are hypotension (MAP less than 80 mm Hg), dilutional hyponatremia, and severe urinary sodium retention (urine sodium less than 5 mEq/l). Some cases may be secondary to infection, acute alcoholic hepatitis, and large-volume paracentesis sans albumin replacement. Other risk factors associated with HRS include decreased free water excretion after water load, elevated plasma renin activity, elevated plasma norepinephrine, elevated urine osmolality, elevated serum potassium, elevated serum urea, creatinine greater than 1.5 mg/dl, and decreased GFR.

Diagnoses

Hepatorenal syndrome is typically a diagnosis of exclusion and primarily depends upon serum creatinine levels. Major criteria, as proposed by the 1996 International Ascites Club, must all be present in order to diagnose HRS and include decreased GFR (creatinine greater than 1.5 mg/dl or 24-hour urine creatinine clearance less than 40 ml/min), no evidence of shock, bacterial infection with fluid loss, treatment with nephrotoxic drugs, lack of improvement in renal function after cessation of diuretics and expansion of plasma volume, proteinuria less than 500 mg/dl, and no evidence of obstructive uropathy or intrinsic parenchymal disorder on ultrasound examination.

Medical and Surgical Treatment

The preferred treatment of hepatorenal syndrome is liver transplantation; most die before an appropriate donor can be obtained. Many medications have been utilized to minimal effect in the treatment of hepatorenal syndrome. Some recent studies have demonstrated efficacious treatment with ornipressin and terlipressin, which act as agonists of vasopressin V1 receptors in the splanchnic circulation. The administration of low-dose dopamine and misoprostol have not been noted to have much effect in treatment. Peritoneovenous shunting has been suggested as a possible treatment for type 2 HRS, but study data are limited.

Metabolic Hepatic Disease

There are 3 genetic metabolic diseases with the liver as a primary target organ: hereditary hemochromatosis, Wilson disease, and alpha 1-antitrypsin deficiency. Alpha 1-antitrypsin deficiency is defined as "a common inherited disorder associated with retention of the liver-produced protein alpha 1-antitrypsin in the liver and low levels of alpha 1-antitrypsin in the serum." Hereditary hemochromatosis is defined as "an inherited disorder of iron metabolism that leads to progressive, parenchymal, cellular iron overload in many tissues of the body—particularly the liver, pancreas, and heart." Wilson disease is "a genetic disorder in which there is excessive accumulation of copper in the liver and brain because of an inherited defect in the biliary excretion of copper."

Pathophysiology

Chromosome 14 is the location for the gene for alpha 1-AT. A mutation at the location of the protease inhibitor results in a substitution of glutamic acid for lysine 342, which subsequently causes hepatic retention of alpha 1-AT and low levels of plasma alpha 1-AT. The maximum deficiency of alpha 1-AT is linked to a mutation of the Z allele. Alpha 1-AT is synthesized in the endoplasmic reticulum of the hepatocyte; mutations that result in alpha 1-AT deficiency may impair synthesis, export, or the ability to act as an inhibitor of protease.

Clinical Presentation

There is a bimodal occurrence of hepatic disease in alpha 1-AT deficiency, wherein children are affected in the neonatal period or in infancy, and adults may be less commonly affected in later middle life. The clinical presentation in infants or children includes neonatal or infant hepatitis, prolonged cholestasis, and hepatosplenomegaly. 66% of alpha 1-AT-deficient infants have abnormal liver enzymes, with persistent cholestasis exhibited in 10% by age 1. Most adults with alpha 1-AT deficiency demonstrate pulmonary symptoms of COPD, with 80-100% of such patients progressing to emphysema.

Treatment

The only effective treatment in serious and decompensated hepatic disease from alpha 1-AT deficiency is liver transplant. This disorder is the most common reason for liver transplant in children from an inherited disorder. Outcome from liver transplant is excellent and cures the inherited metabolic defect as the recipient's alpha 1-AT phenotype is replaced by the donor's phenotype. Augmentation treatment is the infusion of alpha 1-AT that is derived from purified pooled human plasma. Augmentation treatment may be given weekly, bi-weekly, or monthly, and has been thought to be the mainstay in treating emphysema of alpha 1-AT deficiency, but not in treating the hepatic damage.

Hereditary Hemochromatosis

The C282Y mutation is a missense mutation of the HFE gene on the short arm of chromosome 6. The HFE gene plays a major role in regulating the metabolism of iron. If the mutation is expressed phenotypically, patients demonstrate a pathologic predisposition for the increased absorption of iron in the diet that results in progressive development of cirrhosis, hepatocellular carcinoma, diabetes, and cardiac disease. Studies have demonstrated that the impaired HFE protein does not provide proper information to the villous cells in the small bowel, which leads to erroneous information of iron deficiency.

Causes of Iron Overload

The primary cause of iron overload is hereditary hemochromatosis. Type 1 is HFE-related as C282Y homozygotes, C282Y:H63D compound heterozygotes, and rare alternative HFE mutations. Types 2, 3, and 4 are related to non-HFE mutations. Secondary causes of iron overload include iron-loading anemias with or without blood transfusion, chronic hepatic diseases, hepatitis B, hepatitis C, alcoholic liver disease, non-alcoholic fatty liver disease, porphyria cutanea tarda, iron overload secondary to the diet, various other causes, African iron overload with or without genetic predisposition, neonatal iron overload, aceruloplasminemia, and atransferrinemia. Hereditary hemochromatosis is the most typical Mendelian inherited disorder in Caucasians.

Clinical Presentation

Currently, most patients with hereditary hemochromatosis are not symptomatic and have only abnormal laboratory findings without evidence of abnormal physical findings. The classic triad of hemochromatosis, which is cirrhosis, diabetes, and skin pigmentation ("Bronzed diabetes"), is not manifested in these patients. Symptoms associated with early hemochromatosis are typically nonspecific in nature and include weakness, fatigue, malaise, lethargy, and unintentional weight loss. Arthralgias, loss of libido, and impotence can also be early signs of hemochromatosis. Later in the course of the disease, heavy iron overload results in significant hepatomegaly, abnormal LFTs, skin pigmentation, glucose intolerance, and cardiac symptoms.

Treatment

The initial treatment of hereditary hemochromatosis is as follows: phlebotomy of one unit of blood (500 cc) once or twice weekly based upon tolerance; measure hematocrit and hemoglobin prior to phlebotomy treatment to make sure that the values do not decrease more than 20% of the original value; follow serum ferritin levels at various intervals and hold phlebotomy when serum ferritin is lower than 50 ng/ml; and avoid any supplementation of vitamin C. Maintenance treatment of hereditary hemochromatosis entails phlebotomy about every 2 to 3 months with the goal of keeping serum ferritin levels between 25 and 50 ng/ml.

Wilson Disease

Wilson disease is an inherited disease that is transmitted in an autosomal recessive manner. Patients who are homozygous for Wilson disease will manifest clinical symptoms of the disease. The prevalence of Wilson disease is 1 in 30,000 worldwide. Copper serves as a cofactor for numerous enzymes and proteins and also serves to aid in mobilizing iron stores in tissue. Absorption of copper takes place in the small bowel and is transported to the liver via the portal circulation. Transfer of copper from the liver to the bile is critical in copper homeostasis. The genetic mutation in Wilson disease results in diminished biliary copper excretion with subsequent copper accumulation in the liver.

Clinical Manifestations

The most typical manifestations of Wilson disease are hepatic, pancreatic, and psychiatric. If Wilson disease is not diagnosed or treated, patients will demonstrate hepatic insufficiency, hepatic failure, and neuropsychiatric disease. Asymptomatic Wilson disease is characterized by solitary biochemical abnormalities or by biochemical abnormalities and the presence of Kayser-Fleischer rings. Symptomatic disease has the following characteristics: hepatic disease-chronic active hepatitis, cirrhosis, fulminant hepatitis, neurologic dystonia, dysarthria, tremors, choreiform movements, psychiatric disorders, renal aminoaciduria, nephrocalcinosis, arthropathy and concomitant osteochondritis dissecans, ophthalmologic-Kayser-Fleischer rings, sunflower cataracts, and hematologic manifestations-hemolysis. The clinical manifestations of Wilson disease may be widely variant.

Treatment

The treatment of Wilson disease is drug therapy or liver transplant. Patients who exhibit hepatic insufficiency or chronic active hepatitis (with or without neurologic symptoms) are typically treated with penicillamine or trientine (chelation agents). Penicillamine and trientine are given orally and function to remove copper. Zinc salts, which may be sulfate, gluconate, or acetate preparations, may be given orally and block the absorption of copper from the diet by stimulation of the synthesis of endogenous copper chelating agents such as metallothionein. Zinc salts are typically used in asymptomatic patients or those who cannot tolerate chelation agents.

Primary Sclerosing Cholangitis (PSC)

Primary sclerosing cholangitis is a chronic hepatic disease with cholestasis, inflammation, and fibrosis that involves the intrahepatic and extrahepatic bile ducts and often results in cirrhosis and portal hypertension. The only truly effective treatment for primary sclerosing cholangitis is liver transplant. Primary sclerosing cholangitis is the 4th-leading reason for liver transplants in the United States. Primary sclerosing cholangitis may have numerous causes such as possible genetic factors, environmental antigenic exposure, and a resultant abnormal immunologic mechanism of response to the antigenic exposure. Current theory is that genetically susceptible patients are exposed to an environmental antigen that triggers an abnormal immune reaction, which results in the disease.

Epidemiology and Prognosis

In Western Europe and in the United States, the prevalence of primary sclerosing cholangitis is thought to be 6.3 cases per 100,000 people. 75-90% of patients in the United States with primary sclerosing cholangitis also have inflammatory bowel disease, while the rate of patients in Japan with PSC and inflammatory bowel disease is 23%. 70% of patients with PSC are male with the age of onset of 40 years. PSC is a progressive disease with a median survival of 12 years from time of diagnosis to time of death.

Clinical Presentation

The clinical presentation of primary sclerosing cholangitis can vary widely. The typical symptoms at the initial presentation are fatigue, jaundice, itching, and RUQ pain. Some patients will exhibit symptoms that are similar to acute hepatitis. Febrile cholangitis episodes that recur are demonstrated in 10-15% of patients with primary sclerosing cholangitis. The physical examination often demonstrates jaundice, weight loss, and excoriations from pruritus. Enlargement of the liver is typical. Enlargement of the spleen is found on examination in 33% of patients. Progressive disease exhibits signs of hepatic failure such as spider angiomata, ascites, and muscular atrophy

Complications

The frequency of cholangitis and cholelithiasis is much higher in patients with primary sclerosing cholangitis. The presence of chronic cholelithiasis will result in steatorrhea, deficiency in fat-soluble vitamins (A, D, E, and K), osteoporosis as a result of metabolic bone disease, and malnutrition and weight loss from caloric loss. There is a 6-30% increased risk of cholangiocarcinoma in patients who have primary sclerosing cholangitis. The symptoms of increasing jaundice, itching, or unintentional weight loss may suggest stricture or cholangiocarcinoma in patients with PSC. Significant strictures are exhibited in 20% of patients with PSC.

Differential Diagnoses

The differential diagnoses for primary sclerosing cholangitis include inherited diseases such as Caroli disease and choledochal cysts, as well as the development of secondary cholangiopathy as seen in systemic lupus, rheumatoid arthritis, and systemic sclerosis. Secondary cholangiopathy may also be noted in infiltrative disorders like mediastinal fibrosis, Riedel thyroiditis, eosinophilic cholangitis, and histiocytosis X. Other diseases to rule out include vascular injuries of the abdomen, acalculous cholecystitis, autoimmune hepatitis, strictures of the bile ducts, tumors of the bile ducts, biliary obstruction, biliary trauma, cholangiocarcinoma, cholangitis, choledocholithiasis, papillary tumors, and primary biliary cirrhosis.

Treatment and Management

Medical treatment is mainly directed toward relieving symptoms and managing complications in primary sclerosing cholangitis. Immunosuppressant medications as well as chelation and steroids have been utilized in order to try to control the progression of the disease but have not exhibited much benefit. Liver transplant is the only truly effective treatment for PSC. Endoscopic dilatation and possible stent insertions have been utilized to aid in managing cholestasis and have been demonstrated to improve laboratory results, but do little to help with the disease progression. Some recent studies have noted improved survival with the concomitant use of ursodeoxycholic acid and endoscopic dilatation.

Drug-Induced Hepatotoxicity

20-40% of cases of fulminant hepatic failure are secondary to drugs with approximately 900 drugs, herbs, and toxins associated with hepatic injury. 75% of idiosyncratic drug reactions will cause the need for liver transplant or cause death. 2000 cases of acute hepatic failure occur annually in the United States; 50% of such cases are secondary to drugs, with acetaminophen causing 39%, and 13% being secondary to other medications. 2.5% of cases of jaundice and 10% of cases of acute hepatitis are a result of drugs.

Risk Factors

Race can be a risk factor for drug-induced hepatotoxicity; African Americans and Hispanics have a higher rate of susceptibility to INH toxicity. Age is also a risk factor—children have a lower rate of drug-induced hepatotoxicity except in the case of accidental overdose. Elderly patients have a greater risk due to decreased hepatic clearance, drug interactions, decreased hepatic blood flow, etc. Hepatotoxicity is a greater risk in women. Alcohol abuse is a risk factor as alcohol results in hepatic injury and cirrhotic changes that may alter the hepatic metabolism of drugs.

Pathophysiology

Drug-induced hepatotoxicity has numerous possible pathophysiologic mechanisms. Hepatocyte disruption is demonstrated when drugs bind in a covalent manner to the intracellular proteins, which breaks actin and results in rupture of the hepatocyte membrane. Medications that interfere with transport proteins can disrupt the flow of bile, which results in cholestasis. Immunogenic activity results when drugs bind covalently to the P-450 enzyme, which activates T cells and cytokines. Hepatocyte death is the result when drugs cause activation of pre-programmed cell death patterns. Some medications cause mitochondrial disruption by stopping the synthesis of critical factors in ATP synthesis.

Pathological Manifestations

The pathological manifestations of drug-induced hepatotoxicity are as follows: "acute hepatocellular injury, a picture similar to acute viral hepatitis—especially with INH, halothane, diclofenac, and troglitazone; a picture like mononucleosis—especially with phenytoin, sulfonamides, and dapsone; chronic hepatocellular injury—pemoline and methyldopa; massive necrosis—acetaminophen, halothane, and diclofenac; steatosis; macrovesicular steatosis—alcohol, methotrexate, steroids, minocycline, nifedipine, and TPN; microvesicular steatosis—alcohol, valproic acid, tetracycline, and piroxicam; steatohepatitis—amiodarone, synthetic estrogens, and didanosine; acute cholestasis— amoxicillin and clavulanate, erythromycin, and sulindac; chronic cholestasis—chlorpromazine, co-trimoxazole, tetracycline, and ibuprofen; granulomatous hepatitis—carbamazepine, allopurinol, and hydralazine; vascular injury—steroids; neoplasia—contraceptives and anabolic steroids; adenoma—steroids; angiosarcoma—vinyl chloride; and hepatocellular carcinoma—anabolic steroids, aflatoxin, arsenic, and vinyl chloride."

Causality Assessment and Differential Diagnosis

In order to diagnose drug-induced hepatotoxicity, a causality assessment is helpful and includes obtaining a history of every drug used in the past 3 months, including dose, administration method, and use of any other medications such as OTC, herbs, and supplements; a dechallenge, which entails stopping the medication wherein a positive response is a 50% reduction in transaminase levels within 8 days; and maintaining a track record of the medication, which involves documentation of any prior drug reactions. Differential diagnosis includes hepatitis, shock liver, cholecystitis, Budd-Chiari syndrome, alcoholic liver disease, cancer, Wilson, hemochromatosis, and coagulopathies.

Autoimmune Hepatitis

Autoimmune hepatitis is a chronic disease characterized by ongoing inflammation of hepatic cells, necrosis, and progression to cirrhosis. The cause is not known at present time. Autoimmune hepatitis is frequently linked to other autoimmune diseases and serum immune markers, and autoantibodies against hepatic-specific antigens and non-hepatic-specific antigens. Elevated IgG levels are also exhibited. Autoimmune hepatitis is thought to be related to genetic predisposition with exposure to environmental triggers. Genetic factors may include impairment of immunologic autoreactivity; environmental triggers may include stimulation of an autoimmune response against hepatic antigens which results in necrosis, inflammation, and cirrhosis.

Pathophysiology

The hepatic injury associated with autoimmune hepatitis is thought to be via cell-mediated immunologic mechanisms. Abnormal HLA class II on the surface of hepatocytes serves to enhance the exposure of normal components of the hepatic cellular membrane to antigen-presenting cells. Abnormal HLA class II at the hepatocyte surface may be a result of genetic factors, infections with hepatitis A or B or Epstein-Barr virus, and chemicals such as interferon, melatonin, alpha methyldopa, oxyphenisatin, nitrofurantoin, and tienilic acid. Autoantigens that have been implicated that trigger aberrant immunologic responses are asialoglycoprotein receptor and cytochrome mono-oxygenase P-450 IID6.

Epidemiology

Prevalence in Caucasians is estimated to be 0.1-1.2 cases per 100,000 people. In patients with chronic hepatic disease, the frequency of autoimmune hepatitis is 11-23. In the United States, 6% of liver transplants are secondary to autoimmune hepatitis. In Europe, the prevalence of autoimmune hepatitis is 11.6-16.9 cases per 100,000 people and is the reason for 3% of liver transplants. In Japan, the prevalence of autoimmune hepatitis is 0.08-0.015 cases per 100,000 people. 70-80% of cases of autoimmune hepatitis are in women; autoimmune hepatitis may occur in any age group.

Prognosis

The severity of hepatic inflammation will be the determining factor in prognosis. A severe initial presentation, failure to enter remission, and multiple relapses portend poor prognosis. 50% of patients will die in 5 years without treatment; most patients die 10 years after the onset of disease. Steroid treatment has been shown to significantly increase the chances of survival in autoimmune hepatitis. Patients who present with cirrhosis and receive treatment have a 10-year survival rate of 89%; patients who do not have cirrhosis at presentation and receive treatment have a 10-year survival rate of 90%.

Clinical Presentation

The clinical presentation of autoimmune hepatitis can vary significantly. The disease may present as acute hepatitis, chronic hepatitis, cirrhosis, or fulminant hepatic failure. Other presenting symptoms may include fatigue, anorexia, weight loss, changes in behavior, cessation of menstruation, epistaxis, bleeding gums, and bruising after minimal trauma. 33% of patients will present with symptoms of acute hepatitis. Typical symptoms of chronic hepatitis associated with autoimmune hepatitis are fatigue, upper abdominal pain, itching, anorexia, muscle pain, diarrhea, cushingoid features, joint pain, skin rashes, edema, hirsutism, amenorrhea, pleuritic chest pain, and unintentional weight loss.

Other Associated Disorders

Most of the other disorders that are associated with autoimmune hepatitis are also autoimmune in nature. Such associated disorders may include hypersplenism, autoimmune hemolytic anemia, Coombs-positive hemolytic anemia, pernicious anemia, idiopathic thrombocytopenic purpura, eosinophilia, inflammatory bowel disease, celiac disease, rheumatoid arthritis and Felty syndrome, Sjögren syndrome, systemic sclerosis, mixed-connective tissue disease, erythema nodosum, leukocytoclastic vasculitis, proliferative glomerulonephritis, fibrosing alveolitis, pericarditis and myocarditis, febrile panniculitis , lichen planus, and uveitis. Children with autoimmune hepatitis may have associated ulcerative colitis, sclerosing cholangitis, arthritis, vasculitis, glomerulonephritis, diabetes mellitus, polyendocrinopathy, alopecia areata, and thyroiditis. Clinical symptoms in children typically are jaundice, weakness, anorexia, abdominal pain, and pallor.

Nonalcoholic Fatty Liver Disease

Fatty liver disease unrelated to alcohol may simply be solitary fatty liver (steatosis) or may be fatty liver with concomitant inflammation (steatohepatitis). The most likely cause for elevated liver enzymes in the United States is fatty liver disease and is thought to be a result of obesity. Simple steatosis is considered to be a benign condition but nonalcoholic steatohepatitis may go on to become cirrhosis and has an increased risk of hepatocellular carcinoma. Primary risk factors for steatosis and steatohepatitis include obesity, diabetes mellitus, elevated levels of triglycerides, and a high-fat diet.

Pathophysiology and Epidemiology

Fatty liver results in deposition of triglycerides and fats in hepatocytes. Possible reasons for the deposition of triglycerides and fats into hepatocytes include diminished mitochondrial beta-oxidation of fatty acids, elevated level of endogenous fatty acid synthesis or accelerated delivery of fatty acids to the liver, or the impaired incorporation or export of triglycerides in the form of VLDL. 25-35% of the population in the United States has steatosis; routine liver biopsy demonstrates that 1.2-9% will have steatohepatitis. Nonalcoholic liver disease is noted in 80% of obese patients.

Differential Diagnosis

The most typical cause of nonalcoholic fatty liver disease is metabolic syndrome. Metabolic syndrome is caused by type II diabetes, obesity, and/or hypertriglyceridemia. Other causes include medications such as amiodarone, tamoxifen, and methotrexate, alcohol, metabolic disorders such as galactosemia, glycogen storage disease, homocystinuria, tyrosinemia, nutritional issues such as TPN, severe malnutrition, over-nutrition, starvation, and celiac sprue or Wilson disease. Differential diagnosis includes hepatitis (A, B, C, D, or E), autoimmune hepatitis, cirrhosis, alpha 1-AT disease, drug-induced hepatotoxicity, hemochromatosis, hyperthyroidism, hypothyroidism, INH hepatotoxicity, malabsorption, primary biliary cirrhosis, primary sclerosing cholangitis, protein-losing enteropathy, and vitamin A toxicity.

Liver Disease and Pregnancy

Hepatic disease and pregnancy is a unique and challenging situation. Some hepatic diseases are linked to pregnancy while others are unrelated to the pregnancy state. The following are hepatic diseases that are considered to be unique to pregnancy: hyperemesis gravidarum, acute fatty liver of pregnancy, intrahepatic cholestasis of pregnancy, hemolysis, elevated liver enzymes, and low platelets (HELLP) syndrome. Other hepatic diseases that are unrelated to pregnancy but may happen in pregnancy may include acute viral hepatitis, cirrhosis, and portal hypertension.

Hyperemesis Gravidarum

The incidence of hyperemesis gravidarum is 1-20 per 1000 pregnancies and typically happens in the first trimester. A differential diagnosis includes primary morning sickness, gastric ulcers, gastroenteritis, viral hepatitis, pyelonephritis, nephrolithiasis, ovarian torsion, hyperthyroidism, diabetic ketoacidosis, and migraines. No standard diagnostic criteria are currently used for hyperemesis gravidarum but the following are useful: symptoms of recurrent vomiting without identifiable source, starvation evidence with ketonuria, and acute weight loss. 50% of patients demonstrate abnormal liver function tests. Aminotransferase levels, alkaline phosphatase levels, and direct and indirect bilirubin levels are all increased. Serum amylase and lipase are also increased.

Acute Fatty Liver of Pregnancy

Acute fatty liver of pregnancy has a prevalence of 1 in 10,000-15,000 pregnancies and typically happens in the second half of pregnancy. Differential diagnosis includes fulminant viral hepatitis, drug-induced hepatotoxicity, idiopathic cholestasis of pregnancy, adult-onset Reye's syndrome, and HELLP syndrome. Symptoms of acute fatty liver of pregnancy typically are nausea and vomiting, anorexia, lethargy, abdominal pain, ascites, and jaundice. Acute renal failure may happen in 50% of patients and encephalopathy happening in 60%. Liver enzymes and bilirubin are usually elevated. Other typical findings include hypoglycemia, increased ammonia, thrombocytopenia, neutrophilia, coagulopathy, and renal dysfunction.

Intrahepatic Cholestasis of Pregnancy

In the United States, 1-2 in 1000 pregnancies are complicated by intrahepatic cholestasis of pregnancy. It typically happens in the third trimester and usually resolves with delivery. Differential diagnosis includes viral hepatitis, autoimmune hepatitis, primary biliary cirrhosis, and gallstones. The etiology of intrahepatic cholestasis involves numerous factors including genetics, hormones, and exogenous factors; this disorder is secondary to impaired biliary transport that causes saturation of the liver's transport system. Symptoms typically include peripheral itching that progresses to central itching, jaundice (in 10-25% of patients), itching with no rash, and diarrhea or steatorrhea.

HELLP Syndrome

HELLP syndrome is usually a complication of preeclampsia but can happen in the absence of preeclampsia. HELLP syndrome is noted in 1-6 per 1000 pregnancies and in 4-12% of severe cases of preeclampsia. 5-7% of pregnancies develop preeclampsia, which demonstrates hypertension, proteinuria, and edema, and usually happens in the second or the third trimester. 70% of patients with HELLP syndrome exhibit symptoms prior to delivery and 30% have symptoms after delivery.

Differential diagnosis of HELLP syndrome includes hepatitis, pancreatitis, ulcer, appendicitis, gallstones, hepatic hematoma, acute fatty liver of pregnancy, ITP, hemolytic uremic syndrome, and systemic lupus. HELLP syndrome is secondary to a combination of factors that result in hemolysis, hepatic necrosis with increased levels of transaminases, and decreased platelets. Evidence of injury to the endothelial cells and fibrin deposition is noted, which subsequently causes microangiopathic hemolytic anemia with platelet activation and consumption and thrombocytopenia. Fibrin deposition results in hepatic sinusoid obstruction, which causes hemorrhage and ultimately hepatic necrosis. Hepatic necrosis results in increased liver enzymes. Hepatic hemorrhage may progress to hematomas or hepatic capsule tears.

The symptoms of HELLP syndrome include RUQ or epigastric pain, nausea and vomiting, malaise, headache, and occasional visual issues. 20% of patients with HELLP do not demonstrate hypertension; 13% of HELLP patients do not exhibit proteinuria. Typical laboratory parameters to confirm the diagnosis of HELLP include platelets less than 100,000, AST greater than 70 U/l, and LDH greater than 600 U/l. Some studies note that the maternal morbidity will depend upon the degree of platelet decrease. The definitive treatment of HELLP syndrome is delivery; all patients of more than 34 weeks' gestation need to be delivered.

Liver Rupture/Hematoma

The development of a subcapsular hematoma and hepatic capsule rupture is rare and typically occurs in 1 in 40,000 and 1 in 250,000 deliveries, respectively. Hepatic rupture/hematoma usually are the result of preeclampsia, eclampsia, or HELLP syndrome; 30% of cases happen in the postpartum period. Differential diagnosis includes trauma, hepatic adenoma, hemangioma, acute fatty liver of pregnancy, cocaine use, and hepatocellular carcinoma. 75% of hematomas happen in the right lobe of the liver, 11% occur in the left lobe of the liver, and 14% occur in both lobes of the liver.

Pancreas

Acute Pancreatitis

Autodigestion of the pancreas by pancreatic enzymes is the cause of pancreatitis. 80% of the pancreas serves an exocrine function by creating and secreting enzymes that metabolize carbohydrates, fats, and proteins. In the normal pancreas, 15 different forms of digestive enzymes are made and packaged into proenzymes. Trypsin converts proenzymes into active enzymes. Acute pancreatitis is thought to be secondary to a disruption in the elements that area involved in the maintenance of cellular homeostasis. Inflammatory mediators subsequently cause an increase in the vascular permeability in the pancreas, which results in hemorrhage, swelling, and ultimately necrosis.

Etiology

Acute pancreatitis is typically a result of long-term alcohol use or gallstones. 10-30% of the cases of acute pancreatitis are idiopathic in nature. 40% of cases are secondary to gallstones that traverse the bile duct and get stuck at the sphincter of Oddi; risk is inversely proportional to stone size. Alcohol consumption is the cause of 35% of cases. It usually takes 5-15 years of heavy habitual consumption. Some cases of acute pancreatitis, however, may be the result of weekend binge drinking or, rarely, from a single large alcohol load.

Other Causes

Acute pancreatitis secondary to ERCP is the 3rd most typical cause and is responsible for 4% of cases. The risk of developing acute pancreatitis post ERCP is 5%. Trauma to the abdomen causes 1.5% of cases of acute pancreatitis and is usually penetrating in nature; however, blunt abdominal trauma has been shown to precipitate ductal injury via a crush mechanism. Drug-induced cases (2%) of acute pancreatitis have been linked to azathioprine, sulfonamides, sulindac, tetracycline, valproic acid, didanosine, methyldopa, estrogens, furosemide, 6-mercaptopurine, pentamidine, 5-ASA compounds, corticosteroids, and octreotide.

Epidemiology and Prognosis

The incidence of acute pancreatitis in the United States is 40 cases annually per 100,000; worldwide, the incidence is 5-80 cases per 100,000 (highest in the US and in Finland). The age of onset is a result of the etiology: alcohol=39 years, biliary tract=69 years, trauma=66 years, drug-induced=42 years, ERCP=58 years, AIDS-related=31 years, and vasculitic=36 years. Men have a greater incidence of acute pancreatitis usually secondary to alcohol and women typically have acute pancreatitis secondary to biliary tract disease. The overall mortality of acute pancreatitis is 10-15%, with biliary pancreatitis having a higher rate than alcoholic pancreatitis.

Complications

A pseudocyst may develop in acute pancreatitis, which is a collection of pancreatic fluid that becomes walled-off by granulation tissue. Intra-abdominal infections may be a common occurrence in acute pancreatitis. Acute collections of pancreatic fluid, pseudocysts, and pancreatic abscesses can occur and become infected. Typical organisms are *E. coli, Pseudomonas, Staphylococcus, Klebsiella, Proteus, Streptococcus, Enterobacter,* and anaerobes. Sterile pancreatic necrosis may be managed medically, while septic pancreatic necrosis will require percutaneous drainage or open surgical debridement. Other complications include hemorrhage (GI, retroperitoneal, or peritoneal), intestinal obstruction, common bile duct obstruction, fistula, and multisystem organ failure.

Differential Diagnosis

The differential diagnosis for acute pancreatitis includes acute peritonitis, macroamylasemia, macrolipasemia, malabsorption syndromes, perforated viscus, acute mesenteric ischemia, acute respiratory distress syndrome, bacterial pneumonia, cholangitis, cholecystitis, choledocholithiasis, cholelithiasis, chronic pancreatitis, adenocarcinoma of the colon, obstruction of the colon, community-acquired pneumonia, duodenal ulcers, viral gastroenteritis, bacterial gastroenteritis, irritable bowel syndrome, myocardial infarction, cancer of the pancreas, pseudocysts in the pancreas, and viral hepatitis. Acute pancreatitis is typically diagnosed by laboratory studies; diagnostic imaging is only infrequently necessary. Diagnostic laboratory tests include serum amylase and lipase levels; amylase and lipase levels that are 3 times normal are considered to be diagnostic.

Treatment

Intensive supportive care is typically necessary in the treatment of acute pancreatitis. Acute pancreatitis results in significant third-spacing in the retroperitoneum and the intra-abdominal areas; thus, aggressive IV rehydration is imperative. Studies have not noted any specific IV fluid that is superior to another. It is recommended to use aggressive fluid administration to maintain hemodynamic stability. Nutritional support should be started early in patients with moderate to severe acute pancreatitis and may be facilitated by enteral nutrition or by TPN. Antibiotic treatment is indicated for acute pancreatitis that is complicated by septic pancreatic necrosis.

Chronic Pancreatitis

Chronic pancreatitis is defined as "a continuing, chronic, inflammatory process of the pancreas, characterized by irreversible morphologic changes." The chronic inflammatory process results in abdominal pain, impairment of the endocrine function, and impairment of the exocrine function of the pancreas. Chronic pancreatitis differs from acute pancreatitis in that most patients with acute pancreatitis fully recover, while those with chronic pancreatitis suffer irreversible monocytic and lymphocytic inflammation, causing fibrosis and calcification. Some etiologies of chronic pancreatitis are autoimmune pancreatitis, alcoholic chronic pancreatitis, hereditary pancreatitis, cystic fibrosis, idiopathic chronic pancreatitis, and congenital abnormalities such as pancreas divisum.

Prognosis and Complications

The following are factors that are associated with the prognosis of chronic pancreatitis: age at time of diagnosis, tobacco use, continued use of alcohol, and presence of cirrhosis. The survival rate in chronic pancreatitis is 70% at 10 years and 45% at 20 years. The 10-year mortality rate in chronic pancreatitis is 30% with the 20-year mortality being 55%. The risk of pancreatic cancer is 4% at 20 years. The most likely complications of chronic pancreatitis are the development of a pseudocyst and obstruction of the duodenum and of the common bile duct.

Pancreatic Neoplasms

Cancer of the pancreas is the 4th-leading cause of death from cancer in men and in women and is responsible for 6% of all cancer-related deaths. It is extremely hard to diagnose cancer of the pancreas early. 52% of patients will have metastases at time of diagnosis, and 26% of patients have regional disease. The 1-year survival is 24% with the 5-year survival rate being 5%. 80% of pancreatic cancer is adenocarcinoma, with only 2% of tumors in the exocrine pancreas being benign in nature.

Etiology

95% of pancreatic cancers occur in the exocrine pancreas; 75% are located in the head or neck of the pancreas; 15-20% are located in the body of the pancreas; and 5-10% are located in the tail of the pancreas. Studies indicate that 40% of cases are sporadic, 30% are related to smoking, 20% are related to dietary factors, and 5-10% are hereditary. The most typical environmental risk factor is smoking, wherein a 40-pack-year history results in a 5-fold increase in cancer risk. Obesity, diabetes, and chronic pancreatitis also are risk factors.

Epidemiology and Prognosis

The incidence of pancreatic cancer has been stable in men since 1993; however, the incidence of pancreatic cancer has been increasing 0.6% per year in women since 1994. Pancreatic cancer is the 8th leading cause of cancer death in the world. African American men have the highest incidence rate of pancreatic cancer in the United States at 16.2 cases annually per 100,000. Pancreatic cancer is almost always fatal with a median survival time of only 4-6 months. Patients with forms of pancreatic cancer other than adenocarcinoma have a better survival rate.

Clinical Presentation

The typical symptoms associated with early pancreatic cancer are subtle in nature as well as nonspecific and include anorexia, malaise, nausea, fatigue, and mid-epigastric or back pain. The most typical feature in pancreatic cancer is significant unintentional weight loss. A typical symptom is mid-epigastric pain that radiates to the mid-or low-back. Pain that radiates to the back is strongly suggestive of splanchnic nerve plexus involvement with tumor. The weight loss seen in pancreatic cancer may be secondary to cancer cachexia or to malabsorption from impairment of the exocrine function of the pancreas as a result of obstruction of the pancreatic duct from the tumor.

Differential Diagnosis

A differential diagnosis of pancreatic cancer includes abdominal aortic aneurysm, ampullary carcinoma, intestinal ischemia, gastric lymphoma, pancreatic lymphoma, hepatocellular carcinoma, strictures of the bile ducts, tumors of the bile ducts, tumors of the endocrine pancreas, cholangitis, cholecystitis, choledochal cysts, choledocholithiasis, cholelithiasis, duodenal ulcers, cancer of the stomach, gastric ulcers, acute pancreatitis, and chronic pancreatitis. Laboratory studies are generally not very helpful because they tend to be nonspecific. The diagnosis of pancreatic cancer, when clinically suspected, is usually obtained by diagnostic imaging modalities such as CT scan, transcutaneous ultrasound, endoscopic ultrasound, MRI, ERCP, and PET scan.

Treatment

The best means of treatment in pancreatic cancer is surgery. However, chemotherapy and radiation may be utilized as adjuvants or in patients with pancreatic cancer that is inoperable. Factors that may prevent surgical resection are extra-pancreatic disease; vascular involvement of the superior mesenteric artery, the celiac artery, and the hepatic arteries; age; and comorbid disease. Surgical options may include pancreaticoduodenectomy with or without pyloric sparing, total pancreatectomy, and distal pancreatectomy. There are numerous clinical trials that focus on the use of neoadjuvant chemotherapy and radiation for the treatment of pancreatic cancer.

Biliary Tract

Primary Biliary Cirrhosis

Primary biliary cirrhosis is a "chronic and progressive cholestatic disease of the liver." Etiology of primary biliary cirrhosis is not fully understood but theorized to be an autoimmune phenomenon. Primary biliary cirrhosis results in the destruction of the small and medium bile ducts, which results in cholestasis and ultimately end-stage hepatic disease. Primary biliary cirrhosis mainly is seen in women between 40 and 60 years of age. An autoimmune etiology for primary biliary cirrhosis is supported by the following evidence: the presence of increased immunoglobulin levels, a large amount of circulating autoantibodies, granulomas located in the liver and the regional lymph nodes, abnormal B and T lymphocyte regulation, and a strong link with other autoimmune diseases.

Epidemiology

The prevalence of primary biliary cirrhosis is 40.2 cases per 100,000 people with 65.4 cases for women and 12.1 cases for men. The incidence of primary biliary cirrhosis is 2.7 cases per 100,000 people with 4.5 cases for women and 0.7 cases for men. The prevalence of primary biliary cirrhosis is greater in the United Kingdom and in Scandinavia. Disease progression is slower in patients without symptoms who have positive AMA and normal liver profile laboratory values; however, 40-67% will have symptomatic disease progression in 5-7 years.

Clinical Presentation

25% of patients with primary biliary cirrhosis are diagnosed incidentally upon results of laboratory testing. 65% of patients present with an initial symptom of fatigue. The fatigue is often associated with depression and obsessive-compulsive behavior, which is postulated to be a result of sleep disruption (extreme daytime somnolence). 55% of patients with primary biliary cirrhosis experience pruritus, with 10% having severe symptoms. The etiology of the itching exhibited in patients with primary biliary cirrhosis is currently unknown and is not thought to be due to skin deposition of bile acids. 8-17% of patients have RUQ pain.

Treatment

Treatment goals for primary biliary cirrhosis are to delay disease progression and to manage symptoms such as itching, osteoporosis, and sicca syndrome. The only curative measure is liver transplant. Ursodeoxycholic acid is the primary medication utilized to delay the progression of primary biliary cirrhosis. UDCA has been shown to provide an improvement in clinical, biochemical, and histologic parameters in patients with early disease; it is of questionable help in those patients with late disease and cirrhosis. Immunosuppressant drugs have been of benefit, methotrexate, steroids, and cyclosporine have also been noted to be therapeutic.

Pruritus associated with primary biliary cirrhosis can significantly impact the quality of life and can be debilitating. Typically, the first-line treatment is the use of antihistamines; however, antihistamines are to be utilized cautiously in patients with cirrhosis and encephalopathy secondary to sedative properties. Cholestyramine and colestipol have been utilized with success to sequester bile salts but have a delay in onset. Rifampin has been used for patients who do not respond favorably to cholestyramine but the mechanism of action is currently not known. Severe itching that is unresponsive to medical treatment has been treated with plasmapheresis with some measure of success.

GALLSTONES

Gallstones take time to develop and are often not symptomatic. When a gallstone moves into the cystic duct, the flow of bile can be blocked when the gallbladder wall undergoes contraction. As a result, elevated tension in the wall of the gallbladder yields pain that is called biliary colic. If obstruction of the cystic duct persists over several hours, acute cholecystitis will ensue. Choledocholithiasis is the term used to describe the presence of one or more gallstones in the common bile duct. Typically, this is seen when a gallstone or gallstones travel from the gallbladder into the common bile duct.

PATHOPHYSIOLOGY

The formation of gallstones results when concentrations of certain bile substances reach their limit of solubility. Supersaturation then occurs which results in precipitates of crystals that become stuck in mucus in the gallbladder. The resultant gallbladder sludge and crystals then form aggregates that ultimately fuse into gallstones. Cholesterol and calcium bilirubinate are the two main components of gallstones. Most gallstones in the United States are composed of cholesterol (80%). The formation of cholesterol gallstones depends upon how much cholesterol is secreted by hepatocytes in relation to lecithin and bile salts and the amount of concentration and stasis of bile in the gallbladder.

ETIOLOGY

The risk factors for the development of cholesterol gallstones are female gender, European or Native American heritage, and advancing age. Other factors include obesity, pregnancy, gallbladder stasis, medications, and genetics. Metabolic syndrome, high spinal cord injury, TPN administration, extreme dieting, and gastric bypass are also associated with the development of cholesterol gallstones. Certain medications may cause cholesterol gallstones such as estrogens, clofibrate, other lipid-lowering drugs, and somatostatin analogues. 25% of cholesterol gallstones are hereditary in nature as determined from studies of identical and of fraternal twins. A rare hereditary cause of cholesterol gallstones is low phospholipid-associated cholelithiasis syndrome.

OTHER CAUSES

Black pigment gallstones are a result of conditions that have increased heme turnover. Hemolytic disorders that cause black pigment gallstones include sickle cell disease, hereditary spherocytosis, and beta-thalassemia. Cirrhosis results in portal hypertension that subsequently causes enlargement of the spleen. Red blood cells become sequestered in the spleen, which leads to increased heme turnover. 50% of patients with cirrhosis have pigmented gallstones. Brown pigment gallstones form as a result of intraductal stasis and chronic bacterial colonization of the bile. In the United States, brown pigment gallstones are noted in patients with post-op biliary strictures or choledochal cysts.

TREATMENT

Asymptomatic gallstones are typically managed in an expectant manner. Surgery is not indicated unless the gallstones are greater than 2 cm in diameter, a porcelain gallbladder is present, and there is an increased chance of cancer of the gallbladder; or in patients with spinal cord injuries or neuropathies that impact the abdomen and patients with sickle cell anemia. Some patients are at risk from complications of gallstones and may need elective cholecystectomy for asymptomatic gallstones. Such patients may have cirrhosis, portal hypertension, or diabetes; or may be children or candidates for transplant. Most patients with symptomatic gallstones will need surgical intervention.

How to Overcome Test Anxiety

Just the thought of taking a test is enough to make most people a little nervous. A test is an important event that can have a long-term impact on your future, so it's important to take it seriously and it's natural to feel anxious about performing well. But just because anxiety is normal, that doesn't mean that it's helpful in test taking, or that you should simply accept it as part of your life. Anxiety can have a variety of effects. These effects can be mild, like making you feel slightly nervous, or severe, like blocking your ability to focus or remember even a simple detail.

If you experience test anxiety—whether severe or mild—it's important to know how to beat it. To discover this, first you need to understand what causes test anxiety.

Causes of Test Anxiety

While we often think of anxiety as an uncontrollable emotional state, it can actually be caused by simple, practical things. One of the most common causes of test anxiety is that a person does not feel adequately prepared for their test. This feeling can be the result of many different issues such as poor study habits or lack of organization, but the most common culprit is time management. Starting to study too late, failing to organize your study time to cover all of the material, or being distracted while you study will mean that you're not well prepared for the test. This may lead to cramming the night before, which will cause you to be physically and mentally exhausted for the test. Poor time management also contributes to feelings of stress, fear, and hopelessness as you realize you are not well prepared but don't know what to do about it.

Other times, test anxiety is not related to your preparation for the test but comes from unresolved fear. This may be a past failure on a test, or poor performance on tests in general. It may come from comparing yourself to others who seem to be performing better or from the stress of living up to expectations. Anxiety may be driven by fears of the future—how failure on this test would affect your educational and career goals. These fears are often completely irrational, but they can still negatively impact your test performance.

Elements of Test Anxiety

As mentioned earlier, test anxiety is considered to be an emotional state, but it has physical and mental components as well. Sometimes you may not even realize that you are suffering from test anxiety until you notice the physical symptoms. These can include trembling hands, rapid heartbeat, sweating, nausea, and tense muscles. Extreme anxiety may lead to fainting or vomiting. Obviously, any of these symptoms can have a negative impact on testing. It is important to recognize them as soon as they begin to occur so that you can address the problem before it damages your performance.

The mental components of test anxiety include trouble focusing and inability to remember learned information. During a test, your mind is on high alert, which can help you recall information and stay focused for an extended period of time. However, anxiety interferes with your mind's natural processes, causing you to blank out, even on the questions you know well. The strain of testing during anxiety makes it difficult to stay focused, especially on a test that may take several hours. Extreme anxiety can take a huge mental toll, making it difficult not only to recall test information but even to understand the test questions or pull your thoughts together.

Effects of Test Anxiety

Test anxiety is like a disease—if left untreated, it will get progressively worse. Anxiety leads to poor performance, and this reinforces the feelings of fear and failure, which in turn lead to poor performances on subsequent tests. It can grow from a mild nervousness to a crippling condition. If allowed to progress, test anxiety can have a big impact on your schooling, and consequently on your future.

Test anxiety can spread to other parts of your life. Anxiety on tests can become anxiety in any stressful situation, and blanking on a test can turn into panicking in a job situation. But fortunately, you don't have to let anxiety rule your testing and determine your grades. There are a number of relatively simple steps you can take to move past anxiety and function normally on a test and in the rest of life.

Physical Steps for Beating Test Anxiety

While test anxiety is a serious problem, the good news is that it can be overcome. It doesn't have to control your ability to think and remember information. While it may take time, you can begin taking steps today to beat anxiety.

Just as your first hint that you may be struggling with anxiety comes from the physical symptoms, the first step to treating it is also physical. Rest is crucial for having a clear, strong mind. If you are tired, it is much easier to give in to anxiety. But if you establish good sleep habits, your body and mind will be ready to perform optimally, without the strain of exhaustion. Additionally, sleeping well helps you to retain information better, so you're more likely to recall the answers when you see the test questions.

Getting good sleep means more than going to bed on time. It's important to allow your brain time to relax. Take study breaks from time to time so it doesn't get overworked, and don't study right before bed. Take time to rest your mind before trying to rest your body, or you may find it difficult to fall asleep.

Along with sleep, other aspects of physical health are important in preparing for a test. Good nutrition is vital for good brain function. Sugary foods and drinks may give a burst of energy but this burst is followed by a crash, both physically and emotionally. Instead, fuel your body with protein and vitamin-rich foods.

Also, drink plenty of water. Dehydration can lead to headaches and exhaustion, especially if your brain is already under stress from the rigors of the test. Particularly if your test is a long one, drink water during the breaks. And if possible, take an energy-boosting snack to eat between sections.

Along with sleep and diet, a third important part of physical health is exercise. Maintaining a steady workout schedule is helpful, but even taking 5-minute study breaks to walk can help get your blood pumping faster and clear your head. Exercise also releases endorphins, which contribute to a positive feeling and can help combat test anxiety.

When you nurture your physical health, you are also contributing to your mental health. If your body is healthy, your mind is much more likely to be healthy as well. So take time to rest, nourish your body with healthy food and water, and get moving as much as possible. Taking these physical steps will make you stronger and more able to take the mental steps necessary to overcome test anxiety.

Mental Steps for Beating Test Anxiety

Working on the mental side of test anxiety can be more challenging, but as with the physical side, there are clear steps you can take to overcome it. As mentioned earlier, test anxiety often stems from lack of preparation, so the obvious solution is to prepare for the test. Effective studying may be the most important weapon you have for beating test anxiety, but you can and should employ several other mental tools to combat fear.

First, boost your confidence by reminding yourself of past success—tests or projects that you aced. If you're putting as much effort into preparing for this test as you did for those, there's no reason you should expect to fail here. Work hard to prepare; then trust your preparation.

Second, surround yourself with encouraging people. It can be helpful to find a study group, but be sure that the people you're around will encourage a positive attitude. If you spend time with others who are anxious or cynical, this will only contribute to your own anxiety. Look for others who are motivated to study hard from a desire to succeed, not from a fear of failure.

Third, reward yourself. A test is physically and mentally tiring, even without anxiety, and it can be helpful to have something to look forward to. Plan an activity following the test, regardless of the outcome, such as going to a movie or getting ice cream.

When you are taking the test, if you find yourself beginning to feel anxious, remind yourself that you know the material. Visualize successfully completing the test. Then take a few deep, relaxing breaths and return to it. Work through the questions carefully but with confidence, knowing that you are capable of succeeding.

Developing a healthy mental approach to test taking will also aid in other areas of life. Test anxiety affects more than just the actual test—it can be damaging to your mental health and even contribute to depression. It's important to beat test anxiety before it becomes a problem for more than testing.

Study Strategy

Being prepared for the test is necessary to combat anxiety, but what does being prepared look like? You may study for hours on end and still not feel prepared. What you need is a strategy for test prep. The next few pages outline our recommended steps to help you plan out and conquer the challenge of preparation.

Step 1: Scope Out the Test

Learn everything you can about the format (multiple choice, essay, etc.) and what will be on the test. Gather any study materials, course outlines, or sample exams that may be available. Not only will this help you to prepare, but knowing what to expect can help to alleviate test anxiety.

Step 2: Map Out the Material

Look through the textbook or study guide and make note of how many chapters or sections it has. Then divide these over the time you have. For example, if a book has 15 chapters and you have five days to study, you need to cover three chapters each day. Even better, if you have the time, leave an extra day at the end for overall review after you have gone through the material in depth.

If time is limited, you may need to prioritize the material. Look through it and make note of which sections you think you already have a good grasp on, and which need review. While you are studying, skim quickly through the familiar sections and take more time on the challenging parts.

Write out your plan so you don't get lost as you go. Having a written plan also helps you feel more in control of the study, so anxiety is less likely to arise from feeling overwhelmed at the amount to cover.

STEP 3: GATHER YOUR TOOLS

Decide what study method works best for you. Do you prefer to highlight in the book as you study and then go back over the highlighted portions? Or do you type out notes of the important information? Or is it helpful to make flashcards that you can carry with you? Assemble the pens, index cards, highlighters, post-it notes, and any other materials you may need so you won't be distracted by getting up to find things while you study.

If you're having a hard time retaining the information or organizing your notes, experiment with different methods. For example, try color-coding by subject with colored pens, highlighters, or post-it notes. If you learn better by hearing, try recording yourself reading your notes so you can listen while in the car, working out, or simply sitting at your desk. Ask a friend to quiz you from your flashcards, or try teaching someone the material to solidify it in your mind.

STEP 4: CREATE YOUR ENVIRONMENT

It's important to avoid distractions while you study. This includes both the obvious distractions like visitors and the subtle distractions like an uncomfortable chair (or a too-comfortable couch that makes you want to fall asleep). Set up the best study environment possible: good lighting and a comfortable work area. If background music helps you focus, you may want to turn it on, but otherwise keep the room quiet. If you are using a computer to take notes, be sure you don't have any other windows open, especially applications like social media, games, or anything else that could distract you. Silence your phone and turn off notifications. Be sure to keep water close by so you stay hydrated while you study (but avoid unhealthy drinks and snacks).

Also, take into account the best time of day to study. Are you freshest first thing in the morning? Try to set aside some time then to work through the material. Is your mind clearer in the afternoon or evening? Schedule your study session then. Another method is to study at the same time of day that you will take the test, so that your brain gets used to working on the material at that time and will be ready to focus at test time.

STEP 5: STUDY!

Once you have done all the study preparation, it's time to settle into the actual studying. Sit down, take a few moments to settle your mind so you can focus, and begin to follow your study plan. Don't give in to distractions or let yourself procrastinate. This is your time to prepare so you'll be ready to fearlessly approach the test. Make the most of the time and stay focused.

Of course, you don't want to burn out. If you study too long you may find that you're not retaining the information very well. Take regular study breaks. For example, taking five minutes out of every hour to walk briskly, breathing deeply and swinging your arms, can help your mind stay fresh.

As you get to the end of each chapter or section, it's a good idea to do a quick review. Remind yourself of what you learned and work on any difficult parts. When you feel that you've mastered the material, move on to the next part. At the end of your study session, briefly skim through your notes again.

But while review is helpful, cramming last minute is NOT. If at all possible, work ahead so that you won't need to fit all your study into the last day. Cramming overloads your brain with more information than it can process and retain, and your tired mind may struggle to recall even previously learned information when it is overwhelmed with last-minute study. Also, the urgent nature of cramming and the stress placed on your brain contribute to anxiety. You'll be more likely to go to the test feeling unprepared and having trouble thinking clearly.

So don't cram, and don't stay up late before the test, even just to review your notes at a leisurely pace. Your brain needs rest more than it needs to go over the information again. In fact, plan to finish your studies by noon or early afternoon the day before the test. Give your brain the rest of the day to relax or focus on other things, and get a good night's sleep. Then you will be fresh for the test and better able to recall what you've studied.

Step 6: Take a Practice Test

Many courses offer sample tests, either online or in the study materials. This is an excellent resource to check whether you have mastered the material, as well as to prepare for the test format and environment.

Check the test format ahead of time: the number of questions, the type (multiple choice, free response, etc.), and the time limit. Then create a plan for working through them. For example, if you have 30 minutes to take a 60-question test, your limit is 30 seconds per question. Spend less time on the questions you know well so that you can take more time on the difficult ones.

If you have time to take several practice tests, take the first one open book, with no time limit. Work through the questions at your own pace and make sure you fully understand them. Gradually work up to taking a test under test conditions: sit at a desk with all study materials put away and set a timer. Pace yourself to make sure you finish the test with time to spare and go back to check your answers if you have time.

After each test, check your answers. On the questions you missed, be sure you understand why you missed them. Did you misread the question (tests can use tricky wording)? Did you forget the information? Or was it something you hadn't learned? Go back and study any shaky areas that the practice tests reveal.

Taking these tests not only helps with your grade, but also aids in combating test anxiety. If you're already used to the test conditions, you're less likely to worry about it, and working through tests until you're scoring well gives you a confidence boost. Go through the practice tests until you feel comfortable, and then you can go into the test knowing that you're ready for it.

Test Tips

On test day, you should be confident, knowing that you've prepared well and are ready to answer the questions. But aside from preparation, there are several test day strategies you can employ to maximize your performance.

First, as stated before, get a good night's sleep the night before the test (and for several nights before that, if possible). Go into the test with a fresh, alert mind rather than staying up late to study.

Try not to change too much about your normal routine on the day of the test. It's important to eat a nutritious breakfast, but if you normally don't eat breakfast at all, consider eating just a protein bar. If you're a coffee drinker, go ahead and have your normal coffee. Just make sure you time it so that the caffeine doesn't wear off right in the middle of your test. Avoid sugary beverages, and drink enough water to stay hydrated but not so much that you need a restroom break 10 minutes into the test. If your test isn't first thing in the morning, consider going for a walk or doing a light workout before the test to get your blood flowing.

Allow yourself enough time to get ready, and leave for the test with plenty of time to spare so you won't have the anxiety of scrambling to arrive in time. Another reason to be early is to select a good seat. It's helpful to sit away from doors and windows, which can be distracting. Find a good seat, get out your supplies, and settle your mind before the test begins.

When the test begins, start by going over the instructions carefully, even if you already know what to expect. Make sure you avoid any careless mistakes by following the directions.

Then begin working through the questions, pacing yourself as you've practiced. If you're not sure on an answer, don't spend too much time on it, and don't let it shake your confidence. Either skip it and come back later, or eliminate as many wrong answers as possible and guess among the remaining ones. Don't dwell on these questions as you continue—put them out of your mind and focus on what lies ahead.

Be sure to read all of the answer choices, even if you're sure the first one is the right answer. Sometimes you'll find a better one if you keep reading. But don't second-guess yourself if you do immediately know the answer. Your gut instinct is usually right. Don't let test anxiety rob you of the information you know.

If you have time at the end of the test (and if the test format allows), go back and review your answers. Be cautious about changing any, since your first instinct tends to be correct, but make sure you didn't misread any of the questions or accidentally mark the wrong answer choice. Look over any you skipped and make an educated guess.

At the end, leave the test feeling confident. You've done your best, so don't waste time worrying about your performance or wishing you could change anything. Instead, celebrate the successful completion of this test. And finally, use this test to learn how to deal with anxiety even better next time.

Review Video: Test Anxiety
Visit mometrix.com/academy and enter code: 100340

Important Qualification

Not all anxiety is created equal. If your test anxiety is causing major issues in your life beyond the classroom or testing center, or if you are experiencing troubling physical symptoms related to your anxiety, it may be a sign of a serious physiological or psychological condition. If this sounds like your situation, we strongly encourage you to seek professional help.

Online Resources

Due to our efforts to try to keep this book to a manageable length, we've created a link that will give you access to all of your online resources:

mometrix.com/resources719/gastroboard

It's Your Moment, Let's Celebrate It!

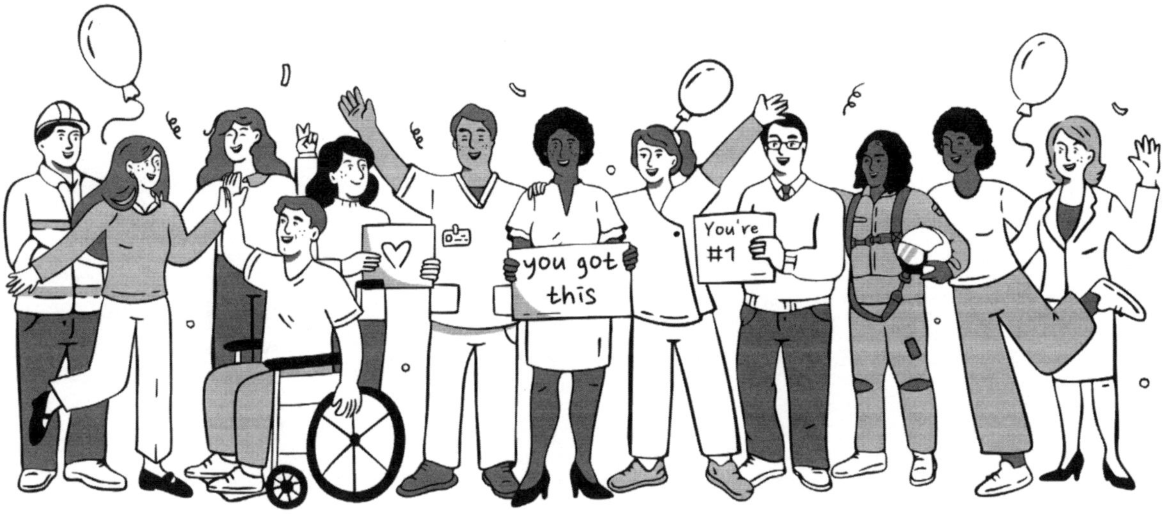

Share your story @mometrixtestpreparation